T0329765

NON-BINARY GENDERS

Navigating Communities, Identities, and Healthcare

Ben Vincent

First published in Great Britain in 2020 by

Policy Press
University of Bristol
1-9 Old Park Hill
Bristol
BS2 8BB
UK
t: +44 (0)117 954 5940
pp-info@bristol.ac.uk
www.policypress.co.uk

British Library Cataloguing in Publication Data
A catalogue record for this book is available from the British Library

ISBN 978-1-4473-5191-7 hardback
ISBN 978-1-4473-5192-4 paperback
ISBN 978-1-4473-5193-1 ePdf
ISBN 978-1-4473-5194-8 ePub

Cover design by Robin Hawes
Cover image by Greg Rakozy on Unsplash
Printed and bound in Great Britain by CMP, Poole
Policy Press uses environmentally responsible print partners

For David Vincent (1955–2012)

Thanks for everything, Dad

Contents

List of figures and tables

Figures

Table

Notes on the author

Ben Vincent (pronouns: they/them) is an academic specialising in transgender studies. Following degrees in biological natural sciences and multi-disciplinary gender studies from the University of Cambridge, they completed a PhD in sociology at the University of Leeds, on which this book is based. As of early 2020 they were a postdoctoral research fellow at the Open University, working on the project ICTA (Integrating Care for Trans Adults). They are a member of the World Professional Association for Transgender Health and former chair of the Gender Identity Research and Education Society. Their first book, *Transgender Health: A Practitioner's Guide to Binary and Non-Binary Trans Patient Care*, was highly commended in the 2019 BMA Medical Book Awards.

Acknowledgements

Since starting the work that would become this book back in 2013, I've received a humbling amount of support and encouragement. I retain only gratitude and warm feelings towards Sally Hines and Ana Manzano, who supervised my doctorate at the University of Leeds. I am grateful to Shannon Kneis of Policy Press for seeing this work through as editor from beginning to end. Huge thanks to those who took a look at various bits of this book as it was being written and resynthesised: Sonja Erikainen, Kit Heyam, Samuel Heyes, Jost Migenda, Ruth Pearce, Kayte Stokoe, S.W. Underwood and Francis Ray White. To Ruth and Sonja in particular, thank you for being among my dearest friends and most inspiring of collaborators. To Meg-John Barker also, thank you for your most valued early career support and friendship, and to Richard Holti for being so accommodating and encouraging of my work. Stuart Lorimer, you're a valued friend and I enjoy every conversation (and drink). To the memory of Harry Harris, who reminds me to be the change I want to see in the world. To Kat and John, of course, for all you've brought to my life. Finally, thanks to my mum, Sally Vincent, for unconditional support and love in all that I do, and to my dad, David Vincent – by making my PhD possible, this book is part of your legacy.

Introduction

Figure 1: Annemarie à Berlin. Annemarie Schwartzenbach, taken by Marianne Breslauer, 1932

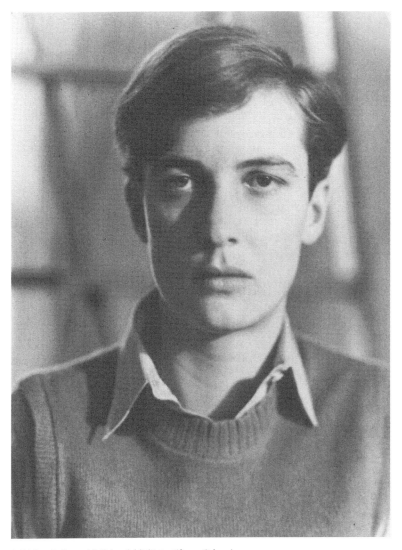

The biggest difficulty with affirming a third-gender category is knowing what that means. (Roughgarden, 2013: 393)

Voices from beyond the gender binary

Gender diverse people have been prompting questions about the nature of gender for as long as they have been recognised. In the 20th-century West at least, trans discourses have been heavily shaped by social/gendered expectations – disciplining not only the possibilities of embodiment and expression, but also identity. In 2002, Joan Nestle, Clare Howell and Riki Wilchins edited a collection comprised of Wilchins' essays and short community pieces, titled *Genderqueer: Voices from Beyond the Sexual Binary*. This was remarkable not only because of its bottom-up centralisation of marginalised voices, but because of the very explicit nature of its central premise: individuals, whose genders are neither male nor female, exist.

In general public and academic contexts, such experiences of gender have been predominantly recognised (where they were at all) as historic and/or non-Western (Herdt, 1993). However, identities outside the gender binary have also been clearly articulated within modern Western contexts, long before non-binary emerged as an umbrella term (for example, Feinberg, 1996). Historians of gender and sexual minorities are commonly confronted with the issue of how we label figures who are positioned as part of queer history. Indeed, it was not only the striking androgyny of Schwartzenbach that inspired me to open this book with her picture, but the photographer Marianne Breslauer's beautiful words about her: 'She was neither a man nor a woman, but an angel, an archangel' (Julienne, 2018). While Schwartzenbach's love of women was known, we can also see a relatability to non-binary through her transgressive gender presentation and how she was seen by others – as captured by Breslauer's images and words. There is a shared history for anyone transgressive of 'normal, proper' gendered or sexual behaviour, whereby their status as men or women could have been symbolically or literally called into question (Trumbach, 1993). This history contributed to the codification of femininity and masculinity with non-heterosexual men and women respectively, even after the lay-conceptualisations of sexual orientation and gender identity had been disentangled.

Was Schwartzenbach non-binary? This is the wrong question to ask. The sexual and gender identities of people from the past cannot be unproblematically housed within newer identity categories, because such categories do more than simply describe who a person may desire, or their self-concept. They are terms that are *embedded* in social context, and relate to temporally and spatially situated discourses. Sexual and gender identity categories in part serve as rallying points for individuals to find and forge communities – accessing and developing connections, and organising to challenge systemic oppressions. Importantly, this understanding of identity categories problematises reading Schwartzenbach as cisgender just as much as non-binary, or transgender. The lack of cultural intelligibility of gender beyond or outside 'male' and 'female' renders historical gender diversity at risk of erasure – as seen in anthropological accounts (such as Jacobs, 1968).

Therefore, I am not trying to insinuate a non-binary 'ownership' of Schwartzenbach when I consider her in relation to the concept of non-binary – her self-conceptualisation in gendered terms is unknowable to us, and I do not believe anyone gains from tribalistic, possessive politics around our queer[1] forebears. Asking 'was Schwartzenbach queer?' is also the wrong question, as it obscures any of a number of potential enquiries behind the wording. 'Did Schwartzenbach specifically identify with the term queer?' – doubtful. 'Was Schwartzenbach a gender or sexual minority?' – yes, but not in a way that can be translated into a singular modern category without the potential to misrepresent or lose something of her experience. 'Is the figure of Schwartzenbach now queer?' – to me, yes, because her choice to live her gendered and sexual life as she did was political and subversive, inspiring a sense of connectedness (for a detailed consideration of the possibilities and limitations of queer(ing) history, see Doan, 2013). The unresolvable ambiguity of Schwartzenbach's image (as opposed, necessarily, to Schwartzenbach in and of herself) *can* be considered inherently politically queer – where queer is taken to be 'about refusal, resistance, indeterminacy, and transgression' (Doan, 2013: 44). This imbues the photograph with potential to resonate with significance for lesbian, trans, non-binary, gender non-conforming, and/or queer-identifying people. In a sense, non-binary people long predate the contemporary non-binary discourse.

The relative lack of research into non-binary identities meant the project this book is based on benefited from considering the factors of greatest relevance to the *collective* non-binary population. The questions which drove the project were:

- How are non-binary people involved with and integrated into queer communities?
- How do non-binary people negotiate existing medical practices?
- What does the emergence of non-binary gender identities imply for queer community organisation and activism?
- What does the emergence of non-binary gender identities imply for trans/queer healthcare?

Taylor and Whittier (1999: 174) state that 'to understand any politicized identity community, it is necessary to analyse the social and political struggle that created the identity'. Queer[2] communities and medical practice were selected as important sites, having interplay with non-binary people's experiences negotiating identity due to precedent from (binary-oriented) transgender narratives of the importance of such contexts (Gagné et al., 1997; Hines, 2007a; Bauer et al., 2009). This is not to say that other avenues of focus – such as experiences in the workplace, of family, youth, old age or education – lack importance. However, I argue that my choices were justified by their extensive and heterogeneous relevance in the attainment of needed or preferred embodiment, social inclusion and legitimacy, through their overarching importance to experiences of navigating disidentification with the assignment made at birth. Community interactions are sites of identity exploration, central sources of affirmation, and grant access to resources if/when negotiating experiences of stigma (Singh et al., 2011). In addition, medical transitions may be critically important to processes of gendered identity negotiation (Levitt and Ippolito, 2014), and transition discourses have affected experiences of transgender communities even for those who do not wish to medically transition (Pearce, 2018). Conceptually, this research took a broadly constructionist approach, as the meanings attributed to personal identity categories, communities, and health services are developed relationally through experience and interaction. This provides the theoretical foundation for the project's orienting framework of symbolic interactionism, which I will return to later. The intelligibility of my research questions and the analysis which will serve to answer them are dependent on consistent and clear use of terminology, which I will now elucidate.

Contextualisation of terminology

Language related to gender identity can be extremely problematic, and difficult to use in a politically sensitive way – especially for those lacking experience with trans communities. Transgender people themselves may still use language that other in-group members consider to be problematic, or as contributing to their oppression. It is also important to recognise that many identity labels are used by different individuals to mean (sometimes subtly) different things, which can complicate communication. These differences can be a result of changes in meanings over time (such as the reclamation of slurs – for example, queer), different national or geographical contexts, political opinions, social backgrounds and the educational experiences that word-users have, shaping how they describe themselves or others. Reflections on naming the self are significant across oppressed groups because of the political implications and ramifications which language use may have, which is context dependent.

It is necessary to recognise that my subsequent unpacking of language is situated, within the context of (British) English as it was in 2019. Many languages use highly similar terms to those that have been constructed in English to describe gender-diverse people, particularly 'transsexual', 'transgender', and 'transvestite'. They may subtly differ, however, or carry context-dependent undertones that are easily missed, especially by those not embedded in a given community and its language. Even native-speaker community members may have a wide range of conceptualisations. While this nomenclature-based reflection obviously does not have the scope for an exhaustive international discussion, examples include how *transgénero* may be used in Spanish differently from 'transgender' in English, and the use of *travesti* or *transformista* in various South American contexts differ markedly both from common English understandings of 'transvestite' and between different national settings, due to culturally situated, differentiated discourses regarding both sex work and medical transitions (Ochoa, 2008). The following discussion is thus descriptive rather than prescriptive, and inevitably cannot reflect the beliefs of all individuals who identify with any of the discussed terminology.

Underscoring virtually all work within or related to gender studies lies the perennially thorny question of how sex and gender are relatively conceptualised. In simple terms, sex has historically been positioned in relation to 'biological' discourses – particularly the chromosomes, genitals and gonads of an organism, and the secondary sexual characteristics and hormone profiles of humans (Fausto-Sterling, 1993). Gender (as used outside grammar) was initially defined by the 'masculine' and 'feminine', particularly in relation to gender roles. However, a strict demarcation has long being problematised through understanding sex as subject to social construction – that is, understandings of what sex *is*, is culturally, spatially, and temporally contingent, and subject to continual renegotiation and emergence between social actors (Butler, 1993). Gender identity has also been framed as a biological phenomenon, emergent from the biomaterial of the mind/brain. While these approaches (sex as *social*, gender as *biological*) come from different epistemological traditions, historical context further underscores how sex, gender and sexuality are all culturally contingent and continually emergent. My approach is not to try and exhaustively fix down a definition of gender, but I favour its imperfect deployment as shorthand for a 'sex/gender system'. This term has a long history, particularly within second-wave feminist epistemology (for example, Harding, 1983). My use here doesn't situate that literature as a theoretical progenitor, though there is common ground. I simply understand this system as comprising those factors which contribute towards how maleness/masculinity/femaleness/femininity are ascribed meaning, by people and through social interactions. Rather than refer to an individual's *sex*, I will always refer to the *assignment made at birth*. This avoids description as sex *or* gender discretely – but performs the cultural act of invoking gender/sex (see Fausto-Sterling, 2019). I reject the argument that sex(/gender) is simply *observed* at birth, as this fails to recognise the act of ascribing meaning to bodies/anatomy/physiology through language as sociocultural. It positions the body as pre-social – the genitals *'are'* male/female, rather than *labelled/codified* as male/female – and so fails to ontologically interrogate sex/gender – as does claiming that a person's assignment at birth simply 'is' their 'sex'. Should discussion of some aspect of sexed/gendered biology be necessary, then using specific, degendered language offers an emancipatory solution. To illustrate with a hypothetical example: a non-binary person may have a hormone profile with a (relatively) high concentration of oestrogen and a low concentration of testosterone (that is, what a clinician might term within a 'female range'). I would reject describing this as a female hormone profile because doing so not only risks the delegitimisation and erasure of their non-binary subjectivity, but essentialises the sex/gender system – and its sociocultural associations – to the material. One could just as easily argue the individual has a 'non-binary hormone profile' (due to the hormone profile belonging to a non-binary person), at risk of confusing an endocrinologist.[3] Precision of terminology can often displace any need for the terms sex or gender altogether (Freeman and López, 2018). Universalising any given piece of anatomy as 'male' or 'female' has significant, negative ramifications not just for gender diverse people, but for the population more broadly.[4] Similarly, the erasure of complexity – by using 'male' and 'female' as shorthand for common clusters of structures (for example, 'male' indicating penis, testes, testosterone, particular body fat distribution and hair growth patterns, XY chromosomes) – flattens the reality of human variation, and is disadvantageous to anyone (trans, intersex, or not) whose combination of traits defies gendered/sexed expectations.

The adjective *transgender* (and its increasingly common shorthand, *trans*) is understood by many to simply refer to any person whose gender identity does not correspond with their assignment at birth.

However, transgender has a multitude of potential interpretations. It can be used to implicitly refer to those who have transitioned or wish to transition from 'one side' of the gender binary to 'the other' – that is, 'binary-oriented'[5] trans men and women (assigned female and male at birth, respectively). Such a transition may be exclusively social, such that gendered clothing choices, name and formal documentation are typically changed to be congruent with the gender the individual identifies with (hereafter, their gender). Transition may also involve medical intervention(s), whereby hormones may be prescribed or otherwise accessed, and/or a range of gender-affirming surgeries may be undertaken to bring the person's embodiment into better alignment with their sense of self.

Over most of the 20th century, trans people were required to transition socially *and* medically, and also to conform to socially dictated standards of hegemonic femininity and masculinity in order to receive any kind of formal legitimisation (Spade, 2006; Stryker, 2008a). This is illustrated in part by media responses to some of the first publicly recognised transgender women – such as Christine Jorgensen, who in 1952 made front-page news in the US with the now-famous headline 'Ex-GI becomes Blonde Beauty'. While the term used to describe Christine at the time was *transsexual*, Virginia Prince was instrumental in popularising the term transgender. She was attempting to differentiate between those who accessed surgery – transsexuals – and those who did not, but still lived and identified with the 'other' (socially intelligible) gender – 'transgenderists' (Prince, 2005). I only use the term transsexual when discussing historical contexts, in which this was the term used by professionals and trans people alike.

Prince's dichotomising model did not stand the test of time. While some individuals certainly do describe themselves as transsexual, many trans people find this term offensive due to its clinical and pathologising overtones. 'Transgenderist' is essentially never encountered. Transgender (or trans) is now often used as an umbrella term (Currah, 2006) that includes a wide range of identifications and presentations. The 'boundaries' of transgender are still debated – for example, some may include those who engage with any cross-gender or transgressive gender presentation (such as cross-dressers, or drag queens and drag kings). Others (sometimes collectively referred to as *transmedicalists*) may resist acknowledging anyone as trans except those who experience *gender dysphoria* – with further debate and disagreement around 'how severe' this 'needs' to be. Dysphoria is commonly characterised as distress or depression in relation to the disjunction between self-conceptualisation and the body, and/or social positionality, though transmedicalists may emphasise the centrality of *embodied* dysphoria. That is, a person experiencing *social* dysphoria alone (discomfort with being positioned as a particular gendered subject, but ambivalence or happiness about the body) would not satisfy a transmedicalist understanding of trans, which positions trans status as a medical condition, and medical transition as the treatment. This narrow understanding of trans-being carries an expectation that 'real' trans people access hormones at the very least and likely also surgery, and those who do not are merely 'trans trenders' (Schmitt, 2013; Garrison, 2018).

For the purposes of this work, I use *transgender* and *trans* as synonymous umbrella terms in reference to individuals whose gender identities do not correspond with how they were assigned at birth. This therefore includes individuals who identify within the gender binary or outside it (binary-oriented and non-binary identifications), but not drag performers or cross-dressers per se. While a drag artist or cross-dresser may also potentially be trans, cultural acts of gender transgression do not in and of themselves position one under the trans umbrella, as I use it. This is also reflective of the fact that homogenising trans identities as inherently transgressive risks oversimplification and erasure.

It seems to follow from this definition that all non-binary people are therefore trans, because non-binary does not correspond to any culturally possible assignment made at birth. As a rule of thumb this works, with the caveat of not imposing any label on specific individuals. Indeed, much of this book's analysis is undertaken on the basis that non-binary is under the trans umbrella, and all except one of the 18 participants in this project explicitly identified as trans. However, it is a point of real significance that not all non-binary people *identify as* trans.[6] This tension is not caused solely by a politics of respect, but by a refusal to gloss over the broad variation between non-binary people. From this the question follows: as it relates to non-binary, how 'should' trans be used? One ontological approach to the meaning/purpose of trans is to describe people for whom a particular phenomenon or state of being is 'true'. Having a gender identity which does not correspond with the assignment made at birth might be the most intuitive and inclusive defining phenomenon, yet transmedicalists would claim the defining phenomenon must be whether someone experiences gender dysphoria (maybe specifically related to the body, or of a particular severity so as to receive diagnosis). Neither of these things – gender modality,[7] or whether negative feelings constitute dysphoria – are always straightforwardly known, and framing either as a binary (cis/trans, dysphoric/not dysphoric) would also be fantastic oversimplification.

A second ontological approach is to use trans only in reference to those who deploy the term as a self-descriptor – who *identify* as trans. Defining transness independently of identity arguably denies agency, and may flatten important nuances with regard to gendered subjectivity. An example of this problem manifesting (without even adding non-binary to the mix) would be a person who has transitioned, but who would refuse to answer any question in a way which would position them *as* trans. That their identity does not incorporate transness even while they have rejected(/corrected) their assignment at birth further troubles our ability to understand populations using a zero-sum logic of 'not-trans-identified-equals-cis'. Terminology such as 'man/woman with a trans history' is sometimes used.[8] This fosters complexity by rejecting an essentialised approach to transness, troubling any attempts to make generalisations about the 'nature' of transness while still capturing an empirical dimension. This may be deeply relevant in certain contexts, such as accessing medical services. Care must be taken however not to 'leave behind' people who have experiential connection to gender diversity but without a trans identity – such as the person with a trans history in the above example, or non-binary, non-trans-identifying people.

Rather than attempt to 'solve' the issue of different relationships with transness among non-binary people, I believe there is value in considering and exploring how and why gender diversity is experienced and navigated in relation to different language. For example, why may people with similar material experiences (assignment at birth, relationship with dysphoria, desires regarding transition, experiences with community and so on) identify differently, and people with different material experiences identify similarly? These are questions beyond the scope of this work. My experience (regarding the research this book is based on, and more broadly) is that it is more common for non-binary people to identify under the trans umbrella rather than outside it (resonating with the findings of the report cited in endnote 6). This is in large part due to the centrality of trans identification relating to dis-identification with birth assignment, shared by binary-oriented and non-binary trans people alike. On this basis, I will be focusing on an understanding of non-binary under a trans umbrella. Non-binary, non-trans identities remain a strikingly under-researched group, though later in the book I offer some theorisation on how a politics of exclusion can feed non-binary-non-trans identification. Indeed, personal understandings of trans, and experiences with communities may contribute greatly to a non-binary person's self-conceptualisation as trans or not.

When referring to any person whose gender identity *does* correspond with their assignment at birth, I will frequently use the term *cisgender* (or *cis*). The usefulness of cis is to decentralise 'not-trans' as default. 'Men' should not communicate (or imply) only cis men, neither should 'women' mean only cis women. This relates to the concept of cisnormativity – which describes social practices which assume all individuals as being cis. This positions cis people as 'normal' – and trans (including non-binary) subjectivities as 'abnormal' in a manner analogous to the erasure of minority sexualities under heteronormativity (Schilt and Westbrook, 2009). That cisnormativity is deeply culturally embedded is particularly obvious in medical contexts, where it is commonly and erroneously assumed that one can always accurately infer a person's physiology from their gendered appearance, or the gender marker on their medical record (Baril and Trevenen, 2014). Cis is a useful tool for naming the majority status rather than leaving 'cisness' to be assumed wherever transness is not explicitly made visible. However, while cis and trans might be defined in such a way to seemingly cover everyone by mutual exclusivity, this flattens complexity that can arise in the negotiation or experience of a gendered identity. A deeper interrogation of the scope of these terms is beyond this introduction. As the meaning of cis and trans both depend on the relationship between a person's gender and their assignment at birth (gender modality), more complex or uncertain answers cannot be assimilated into the cis/trans binary. In short, cis and trans can be very effective indicators of meaning, but cannot fully capture the possibilities of gendered experience. From some non-binary perspectives this may be another binarising frame within which one does not necessarily fit (Barker and Iantaffi, 2019).

Recognising and challenging cisnormativity encourages a reflexive use of written language in relation to gender. Thus, if referring to an infant observed at birth to possess a phallus, declaring that the infant was 'born male' can be problematised[9] due to naturalising and essentialising gender to the genitals. This can be avoided by describing the infant as *assigned male (or female) at birth* – abbreviated AMAB or AFAB respectively. Disentangling assignment on the basis of genitalia from gender identity helps avoid erasing non-binary people. Binary-oriented trans people and non-binary people's existences demonstrate that the system of using genitals as a proxy for later gendered subjectivity is fundamentally flawed. Yet, this doesn't even take into account embodiment which falls outside the sex/gender binary. Recognising physiological/genetic variations (none of which can be readily dichotomised) as *intersex* is fundamentally separable from non-binary, even while embodiment and identity inform each other, and one's experiences of oneself and the social world. Further, it is vital not to erase the political specificity of intersex by conflating with trans and/or non-binary experiences, due to the specific vulnerabilities and struggles faced by some due to their intersex status, and never by *endosex* (not intersex) trans people (Carpenter, 2018). Of particular note are non-consensual infant genital surgeries, and efforts made to hide these from those who have experienced them (Hupf, 2015). Some non-binary people may make the argument they were always non-binary because that is what they *are*, erased by language insisting that one is 'born male/female'. While my use of the term non-binary does not subsume intersex people, intersex people may, of course, also be trans and/or non-binary.

Prior to the cultural rise of *non-binary* as an identity category, individuals who did not identify as (exclusively) male or female might have used *genderqueer*. The foundation for this identity category was laid by transgressive trans activists of the early 1990s; however, the earliest known usage of the word was by Riki Wilchins in 1995:

> The fight against gender oppression...[is] about <u>all</u> of us who are genderqueer: diesel dykes and stone butches, leatherqueens and radical fairies, nelly fags, crossdressers, intersexed, transexuals [sic], transvestites, transgendered,[10] transgressively gendered, and those of us whose gender expressions are so complex they haven't even been named yet. More than that, it's about the gender oppression which affects <u>everyone</u> [...] But maybe we genderqueers feel it most keenly, because it hits us each time we walk out the front door openly and proudly. (Wilchins, 1995: 4, emphasis original)

Here, it is clear that genderqueer is being deployed broadly, to highlight visible transgression of gender norms. Some contemporary readings of genderqueer may intimate a particularly presentation-focused, transgression-oriented reading when compared to non-binary, yet these terms may also be sometimes used synonymously. Marilyn Roxie, who co-ran a blog dedicated to exploring the relationship between non-binary and genderqueer wrote in 2011 that 'the usage of genderqueer may be shifting away from being used as an umbrella term in favour of non-binary when used in reference to identities rather than expression only' (Roxie, 2011), such that an arguable difference between non-binary and genderqueer is/was the use of the latter with regard to gender non-conforming expression without necessarily implying an identity that is neither male nor female. Roxie frames the distinction between the terms as '**non-binary** refers to gender that is not binary (not man nor woman) and **genderqueer** refers to gender that is queer (non-normative)' (2011, emphasis original), which remains a helpful rule-of-thumb. An important caveat (which will be explored further in Chapter 4) is the possibility of identification as a non-binary woman or man. While notable as a cultural predecessor to non-binary, I use the term only to echo where an individual has explicitly self-identified as such, to avoid unintended discursive implications.

Being non-binary does not imply whether an individual experiences gender dysphoria or not, nor whether they wish to access (are accessing, or have accessed) hormones or surgeries. Non-binary people may identify as part of an explicit third gender category. This may be static, or changeable – associated with being genderfluid. An agender or neutrois identity expresses an absence of gender, or the presence of a neutral gender. Some may be bigender, where one identifies as male (or more male) some of the time and female (or more female) at other times.[11] Demiboy/demigirl may be used by people who identify partly as male, or female respectively. Many more community-recognised identity labels exist; however, it is not possible to give an exhaustive account, not least because of continual evolution. Any attempt at formal codification would be dated as soon as published. From this alone, one can see that non-binary gender identities are collectively rich in complexity.

Non-binary medical encounters

It is important to clarify some terms that relate to the discussion of (UK-specific) medical contexts to contextualise the participant healthcare interactions which comprise a significant subject of analysis. First are the different systems of care available. The majority of medical ailments are addressed by an individual's general practitioner (GP) – a primary care physician. Secondary care refers to specialised physicians in hospital contexts to whom one may be referred by a GP in order to address more specialised healthcare needs. Tertiary care is also specialised, and is also associated with referral from primary (or secondary) care physicians. The main difference from secondary care is that it is provided in specialised centres. Gender identity clinics (GICs)[12] fall under tertiary care – these are the medical centres where individuals are referred to receive a formal diagnosis of gender dysphoria, and access to gender-affirming hormones and surgeries.

GICs are part of the National Health Service (NHS), and historically required referral from a GP. The service specifications of 2018 (NHS England, 2018) introduced self-referral, already available to those accessing gender-affirming healthcare privately.[13] Those who can afford it may access private care while remaining on an NHS waiting list, as the average wait for a first appointment in England or Scotland is over two years (Vincent, 2018a), and continuing to rise significantly. Private access to hormone replacement therapy (HRT) is considerably more common than private surgery, due to the latter's prohibitive costs.

In relation to non-binary health needs, medical practice can be conceptually divided into those services which are related to a gender transition, and those which are not. Being non-binary may affect access to, and experiences of, medical services beyond those directly related to gender transition. On the one hand, there are areas of medicine that are significantly cisnormatively gendered, such as sexual health or obstetrics. On the other hand, there is also the potential for gendered assumptions to affect the doctor-patient interaction in any context no matter how mundane, or unrelated to gendered medicine itself (for example, a broken arm).

Due to the lack of intelligibility of non-binary gender identities, non-binary people often experience misgendering – where an erroneous gender is attributed to them. Gendered interactions may be made confidently (yet wrongly) when an individual is read in binary terms, or be navigated awkwardly or insensitively if an individual has an androgynous presentation. In the context of primary care, a lack of non-binary cultural intelligibility and cultural competence (Betancourt and Green, 2007) among practitioners may produce problematic experiences even when attempting to access services where gender would be expected to have minimal relevance. Accessing gendered medical services can necessitate a process of disclosing trans/non-binary status, in order to navigate symbolically ascribed disjunctions made by the physician between a patient's appearance and their medical needs – such as convincing staff that someone who 'sounds and looks like a man', with a 'male name', may need a cervical smear test.

It is important to note that experiences of primary, secondary and tertiary care do not necessarily demarcate neatly. The maintenance of GIC-associated, gender-affirming medicine (such as blood tests and hormone prescriptions) is transferred back to primary care after assessment and 'diagnosis' – termed shared care. Medical records and administration, such as notes on medical files and name or title changes, are theoretically shared between all sites of medical care (such as the GP's practice and the GIC) via a summary care record (SCR). This holds a patient's details in a central database, allowing their data to be accessed by any NHS site where consultation or treatment may be provided. Access to SCRs by doctors is not necessarily guaranteed, and concerns with patient confidentiality have been raised by medical practitioners (Devlin, 2010).

Further, the views that non-binary people have of medical practice may not be clearly differentiated between primary, secondary and tertiary contexts. This is particularly the case for anyone who does not have first-hand experience of accessing a GIC, as lack of experience navigating 'the system' may mean their view of doctors is general. However, the *expectations* held of doctors in different contexts can be meaningfully demarcated. For example, expectations of knowledge can be separated from expectations for respectful conduct. Thus, so can expectations of primary, secondary and tertiary care, because it is reasonable and common for higher standards of (particular aspects) of trans-related knowledge to be expected in a GIC context.

Chapter outlines

Chapter 1 maps out the scholastic terrain relevant to a sociological consideration of non-binary gender identities. This is divided into three main areas. The first of these covers the relationship between gender diversity and medical practice, and contextualises this relationship with subsections on the early-modern history of trans medicine, mid-to-late 20th-century complexification of trans medical practice together with a growing sociological examination of trans medicine, and the relationship with diagnostic manuals and best practice guidance. The second area re-examines older sociological research which didn't have the specific concept of non-binary, but acknowledged and engaged with people and identities (though often only implicitly) that challenged the gender binary. In essence, this will be a review of transgender studies through a non-binary lens. This touches on the early anthropological awareness of non-Western gender paradigms, and community-based genderqueer discourses of the 1990s, but for the most part draws out what I would frame in contemporary terms as the non-binary dimensions of earlier predominantly or presumptively binarised trans scholarship. The literatures covered until this point were largely written prior to the emergence of contemporary non-binary discourses, but the third section covers interdisciplinary, 21st century recognition of non-binary people. I particularly review the range of highly specific and explicitly non-binary focused material published within the last three years, updating this book from the thesis it grew out of.

Chapter 2 continues by covering the methodological details of the project, including an autoethnographic reflection on my own relationship with gender identity – which is continually being (re) negotiated, but was significantly reshaped in the course of conducting the research reported in this book. More broadly the chapter addresses how methods were chosen, adapted and executed, in addition to the management of ethics, rapport, recruitment and analysis. Such space is afforded to methodology because of my stance that how we produce knowledge (conceptually and practically) is intimately entwined with the subject matter – attempting to cleave one from the other would limit how the project may be holistically understood. Further, my deployment of a longitudinal, multi-method approach incorporated novel elements that justify fuller elucidation and justification.

Chapters 3 to 6 are structured in relation to themes within the data. Chapter 3 considers the theme of instability and insecurity with regard to a non-binary gender identity, with particular reference to notions of 'not feeling trans enough to be trans'. Non-binary people described the vulnerability and difficulty of situating themselves under the trans umbrella when not accessing medical interventions. This could be individuals who sought or desired interventions and were either on a GIC waiting list or put off from attempting access due to perceived non-binary specific barriers, or those who did not wish to access medical services. I argue that the medicalised and pathologised history of trans discourse leaves 'trans as condition' (Pearce, 2018) as a master discourse to be resisted, producing insecurity even as individuals readily adopt a worldview that rejects essentialism of dysphoria or interventions when it pertains to other people.

Chapter 4 looks at aspects of non-binary experiences over time. With particular consideration of different experiences of identity negotiation, I reflect on the rationales of some participants coming out as non-binary, but then later self-conceptualising as a binary-oriented trans person – in other words, a non-binary person shifting instead to situating themselves as a man or woman. For others there was the opposite experience, coming out as a trans man or woman in such a way to cross but not step outside the gender binary, later reframing themselves as non-binary. These processes not only speak to how access to discourses and medical interventions have interplay with possible 'identity movement' during a given time for a given person, but how access – to communities and/or medicine – can open alternative gendered futures. I use the concept of liminality to explore non-binary articulations of 'being in-between' before finishing the chapter with a consideration of space, articulating for recognising the role of communities that may not be typically situated as LGBTQ per se, as offering space for non-binary identity negotiation.

Chapters 5 and 6 function as a relatively tight pairing, with attention focused on participant accounts of medical practice. Chapter 5 scrutinises accounts of non-transition-oriented medical care, mostly primary care with some experiences of secondary care services. However, the process of referral to a GIC, which is primary care based, and cross-care experiences of administration are also addressed here. Chapter 6 looks into gender-affirming medical interventions, the vast majority of which occurred in the context of NHS GICs (although some private practice and non-UK examples are also discussed). The book concludes by considering what systemic improvements may be made to queer communities and medical provisions, to allow the heterogeneity of non-binary identifying people to feel legitimised in their identities, and have equal access and experience of services. In order to optimise such recommendations, the limitations of this study and future necessary directions of enquiry are considered.

Notes

[1] 'Queer' gets used in a multitude of different yet overlapping ways. It has been a simple substitution for gay and/or lesbian (related to an activist history of slur reclamation), an umbrella term for gender and sexual minorities, and an explicit rejection of the 'true' knowability of self, or of fixed/stable categories (thereby becoming a distinct but leaky category that resists definition). It may also be used to point towards *people who queer* – highlighting, as a verb, subversive and ongoing action. In this instance I'm trying to capture a sense of historic gender and sexual minorities who were knowable enough to be known, which would almost unavoidably have been politicised as transgressive.

[2] In contrast to the earlier context, here I use 'queer' as an umbrella term for any and all communities organised for gender and sexual minority populations.

[3] Which, more seriously, is a significant problem as medical professionals for the most part depend on deeply insufficient language and ciscentric conceptualisations when providing trans (including non-binary) healthcare, contributing to an inhospitable environment for trans/non-binary service users even where the intent is quite the opposite.

[4] For example, stigma surrounding infertility ('failure of man/womanhood'), the generation of medical screening invitations on the basis of 'gender marker' rather than an individual's anatomy, or bullying and ostracisation related to secondary sexual characteristics such as body hair and fat distribution.

[5] I use 'binary-oriented' throughout, rather than simply 'binary' (versus non-binary) trans to draw attention to the limited and constructed nature of the gender binary,

and that experiencing gender identity in relation to manhood or womanhood does not imply 'buying into' gender stereotypes, or that an individual lacks recognition of the problems with the gender binary as a system of social organisation. Individuals are 'made sense of' by others *relative* to the gender binary – they do not comprise the binary itself. Further, 'binary versus non-binary' flattens and simplifies how people can relate to the gender binary, bringing into being a problematic 'non-binary/binary binary'. My thanks to Sam Hope for useful discussions regarding this area.

6 A 2016 report by the Scottish Trans Equality Network on non-binary people's experiences in the UK showed 65 per cent of respondents identified as trans while 15 per cent did not, with 20 per cent unsure (Valentine, 2016c).

7 This is a new concept coined by Florence Ashley (2021, forthcoming), used to refer to how a person's gender identity stands *in relation* to their assignment at birth. The most common gender modalities are therefore cis and trans. The concept is useful, first for clarifying how cis/trans status is different and differentiable from a person's gender identity in and of itself. Second, it resists the construction of a cis/trans binary, that can particularly fail people negotiating their relationship with their gender, or otherwise experiencing gender complexity.

8 Analogous to how the descriptor 'men who have sex with men' is independent of sexual identity. This is important when trying to assess health and risk effectively, as men may have sex with men in various contexts while identifying as straight (for example, sex work, prison populations).

9 As discussed, this challenges the idea that physiological structures such as the penis are inherently or naturally sexed/gendered, and recognises the inscription of sex/gender onto infants as a cultural act, rather than the naming of a pre-social truth. This also respects trans people who might argue that, as with cis people, their gender was always what it is, but they simply needed to grow up in order to be able to articulate it.

10 'Transgendered' people is a common term within older literature, and is now critiqued by many community voices on the basis that trans is an adjective not a verb (and as nonsensical as referring to a 'gayed' person).

11 Note that being bigender isn't limited to a binary gendered frame and that this is only one example; a person could also be, for example, (more) female some of the time and (more) neutrois some of the time.

12 Also sometimes called GISs – gender identity services. As of September 2018, NHS England released new service specifications for adult gender identity services which altered the nomenclature to 'gender dysphoria clinics', presumably as part of a clinical politics designed to emphasise that *dysphoria* is treated, not an individual's gender identity per se. The original term is used throughout this book primarily due to its greater discursive familiarity.

13 The Sandyford GIC in Glasgow also already allowed for self-referral.

1

Reviewing non-binary: where have we come from?

Medical practitioners and institutions have the social power to determine what is considered sick or healthy, normal or pathological, sane or insane – and thus, often, to transform potentially neutral forms of human difference into unjust and oppressive social hierarchies. (Stryker, 2008a: 36)

Introduction

This chapter situates non-binary gender identities within existing research. I have already addressed the point that non-binary genders can be differentially conceptualised as distinct from, cutting across, or under the trans umbrella. However, it is fair to situate the work done on non-binary genders within transgender studies (in addition to any other fields in which a particular scholar or team works). I characterise this as an inherently interdisciplinary field, with important contributions from scholars of anthropology, medicine, literature, law and sociology, among others. I aim to show how the academic consideration of gender diversity has produced a varied and expanding range of literature that vitally informs the specific consideration of non-binary identities.

Each section of this chapter will approach gender diversity from different disciplinary angles, presenting these literatures roughly chronologically. I begin with a brief recognition of early-modern history, before traversing work on/from medicine and (what we would now term) trans. I then engage with work that critically scrutinises power dynamics within medical practice, and how medical scholarship has framed trans. The majority of this work was prior to the manifestation of the term non-binary as it is now deployed, yet remains a vital prelude to contextualise specific non-binary scholarship, rooted as it is in the clinical and social consideration of gender diversity.

I follow this by engaging with the literature that explicitly recognised 'third gender categories' prior to the cultural shift whereby non-binary began entering more mainstream contexts. This literature is comprised of non-Western or historical analyses, unemphasised parts of older trans research, or consideration of genderqueer or non-gendered identities.

This leads to the 21st-century concept of non-binary genders, and the body of specific or related work that is now emerging. Only the most recent examples of this scholarship recognise non-binary identification as an (umbrella) category in its own right, with older work implicitly illustrating non-binary variation before the term 'non-binary' entered academic or queer community contexts. I aim to look at the literature through a non-binary lens to consider how gender diversity has been scholastically interpreted, and what discursive impacts this may have had on contemporary consideration of trans/non-binary people.

Construction of the transsexual

Historically, the articulation of sexuality was essentialised to the 'truth' of an individual's sex, just as their genitals were. That is, attraction to men was so essentialised to 'femaleness' that anyone AMAB attracted to men had their status *as* a man undermined, and vice versa. Culturally constructed notions of masculinity and femininity also demanded that men performed their gender as 'active', thus acting as sexual penetrators, while to be a woman was constructed as passive/penetrated. Sodomy in and of itself did not pose a challenge to a man's status as male, so long as the man in question was not penetrated. Thus men (rather than boys) who *were* penetrated, and women who penetrated women 'violated the patriarchal code ... such persons were likely to be classified as hermaphrodites and, thus, as biologically deviant. In men, this classification was sometimes understood to be symbolic, but in the case of women, they were likely to be examined by doctors for signs of actual clitoral enlargement' (Trumbach, 1993: 113). This illustrates how early discourses of what we now understand as sexuality, related to the nucleation of non-binary identification. Individuals who conformed to some ideas of gender but transgressed others could be relegated to suspicious or stigmatised gender ambiguity. Older identity categories such as Mollies in the UK and eunuchs in various global contexts can be connected to contemporary identity groups (Vincent and Manzano, 2017). Such groups can be conceived as potentially neither male nor female, rather than as 'deviant men/women' as a cissexist, binary framework would have it. People who challenge a binary gender/sex system have always existed, yet have often been historically erased. I am not suggesting that we simply place a non-binary frame onto the past (as indicated by my discussion of Schwartzenbach in the Introduction). Rather, queer historical analysis is opened up further when a binarised gender/sex assumption is challenged.

Over the 19th century, gender and sexual diversity shifted from the domain of the church to the clinic – from sin to disorder. As attraction to women was essential for one to be considered 'really' male, homosexual men blurred understandings of sex (this predated any conceptual attempts to demarcate sex and gender) – the essential male quality of 'phallus' and 'attraction to men' were in tension. Karl Heinrich Ulrichs was the first to articulate the idea of having 'a female soul trapped in a male body', in reference to men attracted to men (Ulrichs, [1864] 1994). This phrase still gets used today, though is discursively associated with trans womanhood. This underscores how the relationship between sex, gender and sexuality has a significant history that positioned all gender *and sexuality* minorities as occupying a pseudo-distinct category from 'men' and 'women'. Magnus Hirschfeld (1910) coined the term *transvestite* in reference to men wearing 'women's clothing'.[1] However, a clear distinction between men who found pleasure in wearing women's clothing but still identified as men, and individuals who disidentified with their assignment at birth was only to come in the 1940s and 1950s (Ball, 1967). Little attention was paid to AFAB people who lived as men (Cromwell, 1999; Stryker, 2008a).

While Hirschfeld (writing in German) was the first to use the term 'psychic transsexuality' (1923), Cauldwell (1949) was the first to use the term *transsexual* to specifically describe desires for physiological/anatomical change, accompanying cross-gender presentation. The medical construction of 'transsexuality' allowed for the introduction and legitimisation of hormonal and surgical treatment for individuals diagnosed with transsexualism – due in large part to the work of Harry Benjamin (1966), who advocated for such access. While the earliest transsexual surgical procedures were carried out under the supervision of Hirschfeld in Germany – such as Dora Richter in 1930, and Lili Elbe in 1931, these were experimental and not yet more broadly known or accessible. Predating this however was the surgical masculinisation of the genitals of Herman Karl in 1882. His 'change of sex' was officially recognised by the Prussian state (Bullough and Bullough, 1993).

Access to surgical intervention remained extremely limited for many years. This is well illustrated by the experiences of two early pioneers of gender-affirming surgeries – Roberta Cowell and April Ashley. Cowell was the first transsexual woman to receive surgery in the UK, in 1951; however, this was only possible due to a manipulation of the contemporary medical system. Cowell had developed a friendship with Michael Dillon, who was the first trans man to undergo phalloplasty in the UK (Beemyn, 2013). Dillon was a medical student, and agreed to conduct an illegal, secret orchiectomy (removal of the testes) on Cowell – as detailed in a biography by Kennedy (2008). This allowed Cowell to convince a Harley Street doctor that she was intersex, allowing access to the first UK vaginoplasty and a change of birth certificate. This significantly illustrates how the medical establishment at this time, despite some interest in transsexualism as a medical condition, failed to provide recognition unless intersex arguments could be deployed to make claims of the 'truth' of a person's sexed status. Transsexualism was positioned as a mental disorder, with the view of the genitals at birth still being positioned as the ultimate indicator as to the individual's 'real' gender/sex. This is necessary to consider for two reasons. First, embodied, biologically coded evidence was afforded greater discursive value among medical practitioners, which has shaped how trans/non-binary people experience healthcare and identity. Second, whether through strategic deployment of an intersex narrative[2] or not, trans people share a problematic history of being *collectively* relegated to a third gender category. This must be disentangled from non-binary as it is now used.

Transsexualism gained mainstream visibility in 1952, through the media coverage of Christine Jorgensen's transition. Consequently, awareness of the possibility of medical transition began to spread. However, diagnostic categories and criteria were applied such that only the most normative expressions of cross-gender identification were legitimised. For example, when medical research attempted to construct an aetiology of transsexualism, a hierarchical narrative was built such that transsexual people were subcategorised as 'primary' or 'secondary' (Person and Ovesey, 1974a, 1974b). This may be related to the use of 'primary and secondary' conditions in medicine more generally, where a primary condition is defined as an underlying cause, while secondary conditions may constitute treatable symptoms that are only cured through addressing a primary condition (Kinne et al., 2004).

Non-disordered gender complexity: critical evaluation and evolution of medical scholarship

While a slow dissemination of information on transsexualism occurred in the academic medical community from the 1950s onwards (for example, Ball, 1967), the ways in which practitioners' views of gender/sex were culturally ingrained resulted in heavy restrictions in how individuals could express themselves and be found eligible for treatment. This has been considered by Spade (2003, 2006), who emphasised problematic rigidity in accessing gender-affirming services as still present. Spade argued that there is a continued overreliance on medical evaluation and 'expertise',[3] which creates legal difficulties when lobbying for trans equality. In many parts of the world, access to medical care is dependent on one's economic capital. Within a North American context (to name one), ensuring that gender-affirming procedures are covered under insurance policies is often difficult. This means that accessing medical procedures – frequently viewed as evidence for legal recognition – are highly constrained by class, intersecting sharply with race (de Vries, 2015). Health inequality intersections with class and race are apparent transnationally, with differential complex manifestations dependent on national context, healthcare system and many other nuances.

It is argued that trans body narratives are constructed within a context of great pressure to conform to medical expectations (Beauchamp, 2014). It is important to recognise how the interplay between dysphoria and the strategic performance of particular body narratives (in order to access medical services) may affect others who encounter these narratives, be they trans or a trans person's partner (Gamarel et al., 2014). The relationship non-binary people may have with dysphoria as the dominant model for understanding the desire to make changes to embodiment, or how trans community discourses affect non-binary people, necessitate greater exploration. It is reasonable to infer that non-binary individuals will be as heterogeneous as the binary-oriented trans population. Whether specific non-binary identities relate to particular embodied desires – such as being partially masculinised or feminised, or androgynous – also merits exploration. Such non-binary desires may be modulated by interactions with both the queer community and medical practice.

Califia supports the point that trans people often resist medical gatekeeping, in saying 'the gender community has at this point accumulated a lot of folk wisdom about what you need to tell the doctors to get admitted to a gender-reassignment program' (Califia, 2012: 224). Negotiations between gender diverse service users and healthcare providers change and shift over time, not only due to changes in medical policies and how trans/non-binary identities are articulated, but the public reception of non-binary as popular awareness grows. It remains unknown how frequently and to what extent non-binary people wish to access medical services in relation to their gender identities in any generalisable sense. A clinical poster presentation (Gran et al., 2019) stated that 7.1 per cent (152) patients had a non-binary gender identity, out of a total sample of the 2,137 patients who had a first appointment at Charing Cross GIC in London, between May 2017 and January 2019. This is significantly less than the non-binary proportions reported by the non-clinical National LGBT Survey (Government Equalities Office, 2018) and Scottish Trans Alliance survey (Valentine, 2016a). This could be due not just to fewer non-binary people wanting to access treatments, but due to an unknown proportion positioning themselves within the gender binary in the clinical context.

Contemporary trans community concerns regarding medical care are complex and variable. Examples include a lack of inclusion of LGBTQ-specific training within medical degrees (Obedin-Maliver et al., 2011), as well as fears of healthcare inequalities (Bradshaw and Ryan, 2012). Erasure of trans people is discussed in Namaste's work *Invisible Lives* (2000), where erasure is defined as 'how transsexuality is managed in culture and institutions, a condition that ultimately inscribes transsexuality as impossible' (Namaste, 2000: 4–5). This extremity, while impossible in a GIC, may be identifiable at the level of primary care, especially in relation to non-binary gender identities. Bauer et al. (2009) identified two key sites of erasure in relation to trans healthcare – informational and institutional. Informational erasure is defined as 'both the lack of knowledge regarding trans people and trans issues and the assumption that such knowledge does not exist even when it may. It is manifest in research studies, curricula, and textbooks and in the information learned by or readily accessible to health care providers and policy makers' (Bauer et al., 2009: 352). Institutional erasure in contrast is 'a lack of policies that accommodate trans identities or trans bodies' (2009: 354). The literature examining state-approved and regulated transition has almost exclusively examined trans narratives that have been articulated as 'crossing' from one side of the gender binary to the other, with little to no recognition of how gender can be conceived more broadly.

Baril and Trevenen consider how the way a trans identity is articulated affects whether it is legitimised by medical practitioners, and correspondingly whether gender-affirming hormones and/ or surgeries can be accessed. They argue that a hierarchy is created between 'identity troubles' and 'paraphilias' (Baril and Trevenen, 2014: 390), such that claims rooted in decreased distress are given greater legitimacy than increased happiness. Baril and Trevenen recognise how such gatekeeping is part of a larger discourse where medical researchers attempt to create diagnostic hierarchies of 'realness' (such as primary/secondary transsexualism). More specifically, they argue that the legitimisation of trans presentation/expression is based on identity politics, while any intersection between gendered self-conception and *eroticism* is positioned as an illegitimate pathology, which is inherently 'ableist, sex-negative and cisnormative' (2014: 408).

Relevant to this, Foucault (1973: 109) outlined how the medical gaze was able to function as 'no longer the gaze of any observer, but that of a doctor supported and justified by an institution, that of a doctor endowed with the power of decision and intervention'. What is seen and correspondingly judged by that medical gaze is difficult to challenge because of the weight of institutional authority behind it. As medicine has increasingly recognised the role of the patient in negotiating (and resisting) healthcare practices, Singer (2006) highlighted particular factors in evidencing a trans healthcare paradigm shift (Table 1).

While the division of these healthcare models into diametrically opposing factors is inevitably a simplification, these factors can act as signposts for the political positioning of practitioners relative to their trans patients under current criteria. Dewey (2008) has performed sociological health research looking at the interactions between trans patients and their doctors. The research describes a complex interplay whereby trans patients may simultaneously accept/tolerate and resist existing medical knowledge and practices from their physicians. Dewey utilises Hirschkorn's (2006) model of 'knowledge legitimacy' which considers how doctors employ different forms of knowledge. The model conceives of 'technical knowledge', which is legitimised through an appeal to the authority of biomedical research (and its underlying deductive, often positivist epistemology), and 'indeterminate knowledge', which is produced through the practitioner's experiences within the clinic and is socially legitimised by their position of power and expert status. Such knowledges may be transformed into common or everyday knowledge, or positioned as

Table 1: A pathology model versus a trans-health model approach to gender identity

Pathology model	Trans-health model
Normative bodies and genders	Nonstandard bodies and genders
M/F – only two types	Spectrum of body types and genders
Institutional regulation	Harm reduction and advocacy
Gate-keeping (meeting standard criteria)	Informed consent
Experts and providers in control	Peer expertise and community partnering
Pathologization	Self-determination
Gender Identity Disorder	Non-disordered gender complexity

Source: Singer, 2006: 615

exclusively available to professionals. Dewey (2013) has also investigated the challenges of implementing collaborative models of decision making with trans patients. While this US-based study showed medical practitioners as often desirous of collaboration with patients, lack of formal education on gender, together with an absence of institutional support and inconsistency in applying diagnostic guidelines created barriers. While the importance of trust in the client-practitioner relationship was emphasised, this was upset when trans service users felt obliged to present in particular ways as a result of, for example, how diagnostic manuals were sometimes applied.

Healthcare manuals and guidelines

Provision of treatment has historically rested on the characterisation of gender dysphoria as a mental disorder. The *Diagnostic and Statistical Manual of Mental Disorders* (DSM) is a catalogue of diagnosable conditions, and may be used by clinicians for reference when making their diagnoses. The DSM is published by the American Psychiatric Association (APA) but sees application worldwide. In 1980, gender identity entered the DSM-III in two forms – 'transsexualism' and 'gender identity disorder of childhood'. This illustrates how prior to this, for more than thirty years, there existed an uncomfortable tension between trans service users being treated by the medical establishment, yet lacking any formal recognition within healthcare manuals. The fifth edition of 2013 changed gender identity disorder (GID) to gender dysphoria, to reflect 'a change in conceptualization of the disorder's defining features by emphasizing the phenomenon of "gender incongruence" rather than cross gender identification per se' (Lingiardi and McWilliams, 2017: 444). The propositions of gender dysphoria and the creation of separate criteria for children, and adolescents or adults were both accepted. 'Subtyping' on the basis of sexual orientation was also removed.

The *International Classification of Diseases* (ICD – which is maintained by the World Health Organisation) first accommodated 'transvestitism' in ICD-8 in 1965. 'Transsexualism' was first included in ICD-10 in 1990. The 11th edition has moved in a depathologising direction similarly to the DSM by redefining transsexualism as gender incongruence, and housing this under sexual health, rather than mental health. This was adopted by member states at the World Health Assembly in May 2019.

Medical specialists have recognised the tension between the need for service access by trans people and the resultant stigma as trans status is connected to being (mentally) disordered (Bouman et al., 2010; Richards et al., 2015). The renaming of GID was framed as an attempted compromise, due to the fact that 'the healthcare funding systems in many countries are set up in such a way as to make it effectively impossible to assist trans people with hormones and surgeries if they do not have a diagnosis which relates to those interventions' (Richards et al., 2015: 310). There are therefore pragmatic reasons for gender dysphoria to be medically codified so as to allow for maintained healthcare access, even while trans and/or non-binary status are not (and should not be) framed as medical conditions.

In addition to the manuals that describe diagnostic criteria, the World Professional Association for Transgender Health (WPATH) has also produced *Standards of Care* (Coleman et al., 2012). Currently in their seventh edition, these guidelines specifically highlight 'gender-nonconforming' individuals separately from transsexual and transgender people. There is also recognition of individuals who wish to socially transition and/or be recognised as a gender they were not assigned at birth, but do not wish for any medical intervention. However, in practice 'the history of pathologizing trans★ bodies and identities remains prominent' (Hagen and Galupo, 2014: 19). A new, eighth edition was begun in 2018 and is ongoing as of 2020, with new chapters specifically on non-binary identities and eunuchs being included.

Normative and normalising gatekeeping practices can still be found within NHS-governed trans care, such as requirements for psychotherapy before accessing surgical services, and the 'real life experience' (RLE), whereby an individual must live 'full time', articulating their identified gender before particular gender-affirming procedures can be accessed (Bockting, 2008). The RLE has been critiqued (Levine, 2009) due to the essentialist approach to gender that underpins any idea of what it means to 'live as a gender'. Further, surgeons can request evidence of the RLE in an uncodified manner, with the potential to refuse to operate if they are not satisfied. This is a cisnormative and moralistic process, functioning to discipline candidates for surgery in terms of their surgeon's gendered expectations. This poses particular problems for non-binary individuals due to the lack of a culturally intelligible non-binary 'role'. Further, this may force individuals into administrative or social changes they otherwise might not want – such as name or title change (potentially also true in a binary-oriented trans context with unisex names – a name change is still expected) in order to be found 'valid' for surgery. Expressing one's gender identity through presentation and name change may provide significant risks of ridicule, violence or stigmatisation should an individual struggle to be read as cis, which medical interventions may increase the ability to achieve. The RLE was conceived exclusively with normative, binary-oriented trans articulations in mind, from a cisnormative perspective that also assumes all individuals *want* to pass as cis.

It is also important to recognise that information presented in diagnostic and best practice guidelines are nearly exclusively considered by practitioners specialising in transition services, as assessments for transition-related care access are not made in primary healthcare.[4] The vast majority of the literature considering trans healthcare discusses gender-affirming medical services, rather than the healthcare needs and experiences of the trans population more generally. This broader frame of trans and health is under-researched, despite an individual's gender being a critical element within any social interaction. It has been observed that due to the relative ignorance of primary care medical professionals on gender diversity, many trans people find themselves required to undertake the unofficial and unrecognised (and potentially uncomfortable and contentious) task of educating their practitioners (Grant et al., 2011; Hagen and Galupo, 2014).

Gender beyond the binary: earlier discourses

The earliest considerations of gender outside of the Western binary paradigm of male and female were to be found in the field of anthropology (Malinowski, 1927; Lurie, 1953; Jacobs, 1968; Herdt, 1993). However, while gendered expression and identity were recognised as differing from Western organisations and expectations, explanations and analysis were framed in Western terminology, which resulted in the simplification of non-binary gender identities and the loss of nuance in cultural differences. Jacobs, in his analysis of North American 'berdache'[5] gave the definition as 'one who behaves and dresses like a member of the opposite sex' (1968: 25), implying they were analogous with cross-dressers, which is not the case. Kessler and McKenna explain how:

> The Winnebago people were reluctant to discuss their Berdache honestly with white men because the Winnebago could tell that the white men regarded the institution negatively. Reluctance could stem not only from embarrassment at revealing behavior that was being judged by outsiders as immoral, but also from beliefs in the sacredness of the institution and an unwillingness to share this aspect of their culture. (Kessler and McKenna, 1978: 31)

This illustrates how lack of reflexivity and neocolonial attitudes in researchers meant their own relationships with the research went under-interrogated. This methodologically valuable lesson retains its salience in establishing rapport and considering relative social positions when engaging with trans research participants, as recognised in Vidal-Ortiz's (2008) work.

As Hines and Sanger (2010) has summarised, early works that came to be collectively viewed as 'transgender theory' opened alternatives to how trans had been medically constructed, which could be used to challenge the stigma associated with being pathologised. In performing this critical deconstruction, the stage was set for more nuanced investigations of how trans can be understood. One of the earlier pieces of literature which opened discussion on Western non-binary genders (beyond problematic claims of binary-oriented transgender people being 'other than male and female', or discussions centred on sexuality) was Kate Bornstein's *Gender Outlaw* (1994). In addition to discussing non-binary people and providing an academic nucleus for further study (Nestle et al., 2002; Stryker and Whittle, 2006; Bornstein and Bergman, 2010), Bornstein's work also acted as one of the seminal texts in the development of transgender studies. This differed from contemporary literature of the time by not being driven by postmodern theory explicitly, but was rooted in grassroots community voices. Such voices were, however, potentially informed by the postmodernism in queer theory (Nicholson and Seidman, 1995; Rollins and Hirsch, 2003).

In *Gender Outlaw*, Bornstein outlines a clear list of 'social rules of gender' and how non-binary identities challenge or break such statements. By deconstructing the criteria that are commonly used to define individuals as being male or female, permission is created for non-binary (trans) narratives which defied much then-contemporary medical intervention, such as active erasure of an individual's trans history.[6]

Bornstein discusses 'passing'[7] (as male or female) both sympathetically and critically. On the one hand, 'most passing is undertaken in response to the cultural imperative to be one gender or the other. In this case passing becomes the outward manifestation of shame and capitulation. Passing becomes invisibility. Passing becomes lies. Passing becomes self-denial' (Bornstein, 1994: 125). While damning the reification of a compulsory gender binary (or movement between oppressively gendered categories), Bornstein states that to pass is to 'have' one's gender, to be viewed and accepted as one wishes. Thus, 'passing by choice' in order to validate one's sense of self is firmly differentiated from 'enforced passing'.[8] However as one can only pass as man or woman due to the entrenched nature of the gender binary, it is currently impossible for non-binary people to pass as their identified gender, again as a result of the unintelligibility of non-binary as a subject. The potential for such unavoidable erasure to cause minority stress (Hendricks and Testa, 2012; Herman, 2013) in non-binary people places additional emphasis on exploring potentially important modalities of stress management, such as queer communities.

Emergence of trans sociology

Some of the earliest sociological work specifically considering gender diversity was by Devor, who considered the expression of masculinity in women as a direct challenge to the gender binary (Devor, 1987, 1989). The focus of this work was not to consider the gender *identities* of the women involved in the research as potentially neither male nor female; however, Devor's work may be reinterpreted with the benefit of thirty years of further development of transgender studies. Devor assumed that participants '[l]earned from their parents, grandparents, and siblings that the behaviors and attitudes associated with maleness (masculinity) earned one power, respect, and authority while the behaviors and attitudes associated with femaleness (femininity) epitomized weakness, incompetence, and servility' (Devor, 1987: 14–15).

Such a conclusion centres the explanation of gendered behaviour and identification on macrosocial structures. Devor concludes that individuals who are assigned female at birth may adopt masculine coded behaviours and appearances, due to the preferential regard for masculinity under patriarchy. Further, despite some participants expressing significant interest in medical gender transition, they were still positioned exclusively as women within the research. That some participants spoke of 'being a boy/girl' rather than in terms of masculinity/femininity opens the possibility of genderqueer experience: 'I sort of was a dual personality. I still wanted to be a boy and I still wanted to wear jeans and climb trees ... One day ... I decided that I wanted to be a girl that day' (Devor, 1987: 21–2).

Due to how the individual had negotiated masculine behaviours and presentation, this prevented social acceptance when deciding to articulate a feminine presentation, despite being assigned female at birth. This introduced the important dimensions of individual agency, and how microsocial interactions may allow or constrain particular articulations of resistance to gendered hegemony. Being a masculine girl was possible, but going 'back and forth' was not. While clearly related, this early work by Devor did not specifically claim to be studying trans, let alone non-binary people, per se.

Two of the first sociologists to collaborate on an empirical consideration of transgender were Patricia Gagné and Richard Tewksbury. Following Kessler and McKenna, their research considers how 'the institution of gender is taken for granted' (Gagné and Tewksbury, 1998: 81), and that transgender people[9] simultaneously experience pressure to conform to heteronormative expressions of masculinity and femininity, while resisting factors that position assignment at birth as the 'correct' indicator of how their gender should be enacted. Gagné and Tewksbury's work made the claim that most of the participating trans women believed in the 'correctness' of normative gender roles – that men and women 'should' express masculinity and femininity, respectively (Gagné and Tewksbury, 1998), and that transgender people should aim to be indistinguishable from the rest of society (Gagné et al., 1997). While the term transgender was strongly associated with binary-oriented trans men and women, the sample appears to contain individuals who exhibited non-binary articulations of transness, which was explicitly recognised:

> A small number of persons (n = 5) who cross-dressed and had no desire for SRS [sex reassignment surgery] referred to themselves in more politically oriented terms... Their intent is not to 'pass' as women but to challenge the idea that gender is a 'natural' expression of sex and sexuality. This group of five includes one 'radical transgenderist' ... who uses cross-dressing as a means to express feminine aspects of self and to challenge traditional binary conceptualizations of sex, gender, and sexuality... one 'ambigenderist', an individual who lives alternatively as a man and a woman. Depending on how he or she feels, he or she frequently went out 'in between' – as neither a man nor a woman (with long hair, makeup, high heels, tight pants, and a two-day growth of beard). In addition, this group includes three people who self-identified as a 'third gender'. (Gagné et al., 1997: 484)

These participants' experiences of gender were not the subject of further discussion. Gagné and Tewksbury viewed transgender women as outside the (cis)gender binary, by virtue of crossing it. Such a conceptualisation problematically renders all binary-oriented trans people as failing in the authenticity of their gender, on the basis of essentialised physiological factors. Their conclusions that trans women homogeneously believed in the importance of being normative as regards gender expression has also been called into question. Hines (2006: 60) argues that trans assimilation was often 'a contentious political issue', and that 'concerns around assimilating amongst transgender women often diminished through the stages of transition'.

The lack of recognition of (potential) non-binary identification by participants and by researchers may be explained through consideration of Plummer's (1995) analysis of sexual stories. Plummer illustrates how the social context in which a narrative is expressed can limit the ways that narrative may be interpreted. As a result, the increase in trans visibility over the past thirty years has produced a greater potential for individuals to recognise, and to feel able, to explore gender variance. This functions in a manner analogous to how gay 'coming out' narratives became possible, gained visibility and shifted over time (Saxey, 2008). Such possibilities have also depended on the accessibility of queer communities, as 'for narratives to flourish there must be a community to hear; that for communities to hear, there must be stories that weave together their history, their identity, their politics' (Plummer, 1995: 87).

One of the earliest attempts to formulate a 'sociology of transsexualism' was made by Hird, through the discussion of authenticity, performativity, and transgression. Hird specifies how shifts from concerns with 'authenticity' to 'performativity' have been brought about by a rise in sociological analyses, and a decline in an emphasis on psychological approaches to transgender. Hird (2000, 2002) argues that the discipline of psychology, as a natural science, still makes essentialist and positivist assumptions concerning gender, which struggle to 'keep up' with the diverse and expanding articulation of identities. This critique evidences an epistemological shift, with a wide range of possible social scientific analytic frameworks not making claims of the 'realness' of identities, but the importance of recognising different enactments, aspects or interpretations of the self.

In addition to discussing the typologies of authenticity and performativity within transgender studies, Hird also positions 'transgression' as a critical theme, as trans narratives have called into question older views on the relationship between sex and gender. This made the assumption that sex and gender can be differentially defined and demarcated unproblematically, which has been challenged (Fausto-Sterling, 2019). Parallels are drawn between gender and sexuality, usefully illustrating how homosexuality, lesbianism and heterosexuality have all been acknowledged as socially constructed (Ingraham, 1994; Seidman, 1996), as trans people were coming to be understood outside of medical contexts. Hird recognises that within Gagné and Tewksbury's (1998) work, as well as that of Hausman (1995), trans identity negotiation was interactive. This was consistent with sociological consideration of the self, and with personal narratives (Goffman, 1959; Plummer, 1995).

Hines (2007a) specifically acknowledged the significance of trans communities in the production of transgender sociology. This work illustrated the importance of community movements for trans people, in contrast to earlier decades when stigma, together with guidance from doctors, encouraged transsexuals to go 'deep stealth' – sharing their trans history with no one. In focusing on how care is articulated, Hines (2007b) argues that trans social movements not only 'fill in gaps' left by professional services due to lack of provision and effective training, but serve to challenge the efficacy of a system that requires grassroots resistance and support. Care within medical systems was also discussed by Hines' research participants, highlighting feelings that there was a need for greater awareness and training. This raises questions not only over practices of care used by members of non-binary communities, but whether there are concerns (and if so, what) with how medical care is given. Increased recognition of non-binary narratives would serve to assist in the production of a 'politics of difference' (Hines, 2013), a system which encourages interaction between organisations that create policies and minority groups so as to allow for flexible and optimisable treatment of members of those groups.

Hines (2006: 49) has argued that 'a lack of emphasis on particularity[10] within poststructuralist and postmodern theory has led to a homogenous theorisation of transgender'. Trans interviewees in Hines' study rejected an 'essential categorisation' of trans, supporting the movement from an essentialist disease-based model to a sociologically supported identity-based model in clinical practice. However, the conceptualisations of trans held by UK medical professionals have lacked sociological examination, particularly regarding gender beyond the binary. In demonstrating the importance of particularity, Hines (2006: 64) puts forward that a queer sociological framework is key to overcoming limitations within queer approaches to transgender, as this would situate analysis within 'the material and embodied contours of transgender lives'.

In understanding how gendered difference is accommodated into legal systems and social policy, Surya Monro has produced scholarship looking at UK trans politics and citizenship (Monro, 2005a; Monro and Warren, 2004). Further, Monro is among the first to explicitly recognise gender beyond male or female within the sociology of transgender, once again building from, but also critiquing, earlier postmodern theory (Monro, 2005b). Systems of categorisation struggle to be consistent and to grant equal ease of participation, as they 'fail to address the fluid and developmental nature of identity' (Monro, 2003: 442). Monro highlights this using the example of Hijra in India, a non-Western, non-binary gender identity (Nanda, 1990). Further, the significant and specific manner in which intersex citizenship is troubled by the embedding of the gender binary in law and policy is positioned as twofold, due to how the binaries of physical attribution ('male or female genitalia') and identity can both be challenged by intersex. Such work also bridges demarcations between different binary-disrupting experiences (intersex and non-binary) through common problems in relation to equal citizenship.

Diane Richardson has discussed how, through the rise of a neoliberal politics of normalisation, questions are raised about 'what communities and which individuals are becoming *acceptably* visible, as others are being marginalised' (Richardson, 2005: 524, italics original). Analysing neoliberalism recognises how identity politics have interplay with consumption under capitalism – with media discourses subsequently proclaiming the 'transgender tipping point' (Steinmetz, 2014). Earlier work considering sexual citizenship raised the importance of recognising the institutionalisation of heterosexual and male privileges (Richardson, 1998), yet the relationship between sexuality and gender identity meant that a logical extension from such work was how gender identity may limit equal experience of citizenship (Monro and Warren, 2004; Monro, 2005a; Richardson, 2007; Hines, 2013; Monro and Richardson, 2014). Such analyses imply a potential hierarchy of gender diversity, with citizens who normatively integrate, produce and consume possessing greater social capital. This disadvantages non-binary identification under a politics of normalisation, as the unintelligibility (Butler, 1993) of non-binary is inherently transgressive of gender norms.

In highlighting further problems caused by the gender binary's dominance, Monro (2007) has considered challenges to the gender binary through a cross-cultural comparison between India and the UK, in order to support diversity and challenge systemic inequalities. Vidal-Ortiz (2008) importantly recognises how trans narratives have also become considerably more fractured in terms of intersectional considerations such as race and class, though this remains under-researched. These intersectional considerations are an important development since the sociological development of transgender studies, as the methodologies of postmodern approaches and less culturally nuanced natural scientific/medical research collectively failed to fully recognise the heterogeneity of trans experiences. Increased recognition of trans people of colour was an important development within transgender studies (de Vries, 2015),[11] such that analysis of trans embodiment and experience is not reduced to consideration of gender in a vacuum, with no further recognition of additional factors entwined with how gender may be experienced.

Whitley (2013) has considered the negotiation of relational identities among whom he terms 'SOFFAs' – significant others, family members, friend and allies of transgender people. Participants were conceived as 'undoing' and 'redoing' their understandings of gender based on the new embodiments and identities to which SOFFAs were exposed. Tensions between factors such as concern for the trans person they know, anxiety to not offend, and how to be effective in their support were considered in contrast to stigmatisation, which SOFFAs registered from external sources or recognised in themselves. Such work raises the question as to how trans (including non-binary) people conceive and perceive the interactions they have with their friends and loved ones – with regards not only to coming out and any potential transitions, but in the navigation of routine life.

While the vast majority of sociological consideration of gender diversity has focused exclusively on trans men and women, there are examples whereby a diversity of trans narratives beyond the gender binary are acknowledged. Ekins and King (1999) provide a model that accommodates and explores this in writing of a sociology of 'transgendered' bodies. Transition narratives are opened beyond 'male-to-female' or 'female-to-male', but as potentially 'migratory', 'oscillatory', 'erasing' or 'transcending'. Gender beyond male and female is directly referenced via the category of transcending, allowing space for a sociology of non-binary trans bodies. In setting up such a framework, Ekins and King (1999: 600) proposed the next step to be to 'set such a psychobiological focus firmly within the study of social interaction, social situation, social structure and social system', of which medical and queer social experiences play a significant part, supporting this project's lines of enquiry. However, Ekins and King do still draw conclusions which make certain 'binarising' assumptions. For example, they make the argument that '[t]he critique of the binary gender divide and the ideas of gender fluidity and impermanence would seem to rule out surgical and hormonal substituting because of their permanent and binary nature' (Ekins and King, 1999: 597).

This fails to recognise how only particular *combinations* of biological traits are legitimised as normative (such as breasts, vagina, 'feminised' fat distribution, 'female' hair growth patterns). Accessing medical services may result in some biological structures/patterns associated with maleness, and others with femaleness (for example, taking oestrogen and receiving breast implants but retaining the penis and testicles). The motivations for accessing or not accessing surgical and hormonal interventions are heterogeneous and potentially complex. Finally, in ascribing all hormonal and surgical interventions as 'binary in nature', Ekins and King are not recognising how it is only hegemonic gender discourse that is inscribed onto physiology, and that this may be resisted through a deconstruction of sex. For example, the 'breasts' of an AFAB person may be understood as male or non-binary rather than inherently female – a queer possibility if self-concept and agency are empowered in the ascription of meaning to individual, specific bodies. This also grants space for the personal inscription of meaning onto medical interventions.

An important contribution came from Bilodeau (2005), where explicitly non-binary transgender identities were analysed by repurposing the D'Augelli (1994) lifespan model of sexual orientation identity development. This analysis came before most of the larger empirical studies of binary-oriented trans people within sociology, contextualising why a model for understanding sexual orientation was deployed. Great detail was possible by focusing on analysis of two participants, highlighting the negotiation of feminist and trans identities, and anti-essentialist gender identification (such as simultaneous identification as non-binary and as woman). Valuable support is illustrated for the importance of trans communities in the exploration of non-binary identification, and also recognising potential in-group tensions, as one participant suggested that trans women may 'take much of their [male] privilege with them' (Bilodeau, 2005: 42). This echoes the (often abusive) challenges made to trans women by some cisgender radical feminists (Stone, 2006); however, the positionality as an intracommunity tension deserves greater attention.

Differences between individuals' views regarding the gender binary as constructed or essentialised, and the validity of difference between trans narratives has led to problematic hierarchies of 'transness' within some trans communities (Roen, 2002; Schilt and Waszkiewicz, 2006). A key example of this is the phenomenon of transmedicalism, as discussed in the Introduction. An alternative community term (sometimes used pejoratively, and in other contexts claimed as an identity) is 'truscum'. The truscum identity operates a politics of exclusion that judges the experience of dysphoria and binary identification necessary to 'allow' an individual to identify as trans.[12] There is virtually no mention of truscum within the academic literature, further highlighting the space for research into the nuances of trans community tensions, notably the potential for this to be along a deeply unfortunate 'binary versus non-binary' line. Such tensions within trans communities are not new, with accounts of postoperative trans women experiencing social exclusion from transgender women who had not had surgery (Keatley, 2015). Such developments recognise how the internet is an increasingly important site of trans community interactions (Drager, 2012; Pearce, 2012).

Twenty-first-century recognition of non-binary genders

An important earlier investigation into differences between the experiences and identities of binary-oriented and non-binary trans people is an analysis of the 2008 National Transgender Discrimination Survey by Harrison et al. (2012). The data from the 860 respondents who did not identify as men or women[13] was compared with the 5,590 binary-oriented trans respondents who did so identify. A significant observation of the study included the 860 participants being refused medical service at lower rates, but being more likely to avoid seeking professional medical care when sick or injured. It is possible this reflects a greater anxiety in non-binary people of ignorance in medical practitioners concerning their gender identities, but it is also important to recognise the US cultural context within which this research is situated.[14] The non-binary respondents were also more likely to have attempted suicide when compared to the binary-oriented trans population, have higher levels of educational attainment, be more likely to have participated in 'underground or informal economies for income' (Harrison et al., 2012: 22) such as sex work or drug dealing, and were significantly less likely to be white, assigned male at birth or over the age of 45. Such information may be helpful in contextualising the experiences of non-binary communities, as the interactions that people experience (and produce meaning through) will be influenced by demographic membership. Further work has recognised the potential fluidity in non-binary identification. In the UK 2012 Trans Mental Health Survey, McNeil et al. (2012: 6) asked 'Which of the following best describes you?', including the possible answers 'I have a constant and clear non-binary gender identity' and 'I have a variable or fluid non-binary gender identity'. Modelling non-binary in potentially liminal as well as static terms may be beneficial for the operationalisation of data and interpretation of non-binary lived experiences.

The Scottish Trans Equality Network conducted a survey of non-binary people in the UK between July–September 2015, receiving 895 respondents. The survey focused on experiences of using services, experiences of employment and views on legal gender recognition. Multiple reports were produced, oriented to guidance for service providers and employers (Valentine, 2016b), reporting non-binary experiences overall in the UK (Valentine, 2016c), and non-binary experiences of GICs (Valentine, 2016a). Some of the key findings included 11 per cent being refused services due to non-binary status, and 34 per cent being told that a service didn't know enough about non-binary people to help them. Fifty-two per cent never felt comfortable to be out at work, and 88 per cent worried their identity would make the work environment more difficult; 78 per cent would like to change their legal gender on some (14 per cent) or all (64 per cent) documentation.

Another comparably early example of work looking specifically at contemporary narratives of non-binary gender identities has been conducted by Yeadon-Lee (2016). Qualitative analysis was performed of online forums and blog posts that discussed non-binary identification. Analysis of personal negotiations of gender were delineated into two generation categories: younger (age 29 and below) and older (age 30 and above). Within the blogs examined, Yeadon-Lee found evidence that suggested how in some cases the wide array of identity labels that now exists can be a positive resource fostering self-determination, while in others there could be a pressure to 'find the place you fit', and to feel insecurity and uncertainty. Discourses also related back to older binary-oriented trans narratives, with the suggestion that engaging with these narratives aided in interrogation of the internal sense of self, rather than acting to constrain. Yeadon-Lee also discussed how labels could create 'a sense of outsiderness', citing a particular blog writer who said 'I feel like sort of an imposter among non-binaries' (Yeadon-Lee, 2016: 29). Instability and insecurity of identity, and the (re)production of an artificial hierarchy of transness are themes I explore in Chapter 3 in relation to the data produced by this project.

The last several years has seen an upshot in specific attention to non-binary recognition in academic work. This has included valuable reviews of the literature serving to orient and contextualise work on non-binary genders, spanning health contexts (Matsuno and Budge, 2017; Monro, 2019; Vincent, 2019), and more generally (Hegarty et al., 2018). There have also been a small number of explicitly focused edited collections (Richards et al., 2017; Rajunov and Duane, 2019), and a 2019 special edition on non-binary published in the *International Journal of Transgenderism*.[15] There has been a growth of work particularly within transgender health research that has reoriented its use of language in a non-binary-inclusive fashion (for example, Fowler et al., 2018; Grimstad et al., 2018) or wider comparisons of binary-oriented and non-binary trans experiences and needs (Burgwal et al., 2019; Motmans et al., 2019). Since Yeadon-Lee's work, there have been a modest but significant proliferation of interview-based studies with non-binary people.

A brilliant contribution has been made by Rillark Bolton (2019) who has explored non-binary people's use of testosterone. Through interviews with non-binary people, processes of personal navigation and conceptualisation are unpacked that resolve potential tensions between those with a non-male identity, when testosterone is strongly socially coded as a fundamentally male and masculinising substance. While recognising that firmly distinguishing between binary-oriented and non-binary trans experiences can 'in a similar way to the apparent opposition between transsexual and transgender, reiterate a false dichotomy between old/binary/wrong and young/non-binary/right' (Bolton, 2019: 17), the experiences highlighted showed how hormone access can be about a process of unmaking, rather than 'affirming' gender identity. This could mean, for instance, situating oneself as emphatically not a cis woman/female. One participant also articulated 'coming out' not as a process of stepping into an identity category, but rather as 'coming out as a testosterone user' – such that the relationship between accessing a process of embodied change and the expected confession of a suitable identity to justify such interventions are radically reimagined. Drawing on Mol's (1999) work on ontological politics, which contends that social and medical practices do not proceed from, but shape reality, Bolton opens up recognition of non-binary practices and ways of being to potentially reformulate the entirely of the gender/sex system.

Bradford et al. (2018) engaged in a thematic analysis of genderqueer narratives. They highlight important points such as the importance of recognising that 'a genderqueer identity is not mutually exclusive to other identity labels such as male, female, transmasculine and transfeminine' (Bradford et al., 2018, 3–4). It is argued that genderqueer and binary-oriented trans people collectively transgress a 'cisnormative master narrative' of gender, but that genderqueerness further transgresses and disrupts a conceptualisation of transness in medicalised terms that aspires to the production of gendered normality. This draws on Johnson's (2016: 465) concept of transnormativity, which describes 'the specific framework to which transgender people's presentations and experiences are held accountable'. This offers a clear and deployable theorisation of the discourses and structures that can produces hierarchies of legitimacy in how trans and gender diverse people are viewed – by doctors, the general public or other community members. Work that has analysed non-binary identities from a psychoanalytic perspective has constructed related arguments about identity development, experiences of language and visibility, and potential tensions in clinical settings (Losty and O'Connor, 2018).

Of great relevance is the work done by Taylor et al. (2018) who, by also using thematic analysis, explored the experiences of everyday life of non-binary people who had presented at The Laurels GIC in Exeter, UK. The material is limited due to only recruiting eight participants. There can be reluctance to speak openly with researchers based within clinics, due to either anxiety that one could not be candid (else risk being seen as a 'difficult patient' and subsequently impact access to treatment), or a lack of trust that the work would be done sensitively or competently – concerns which are commonly voiced within trans communities (Adams et al., 2017; Tagonist, 2009; Vincent, 2018b) and recognised in the journal article's limitations. Themes were comparable to other emergent work with non-binary people, broadly expressing the difficulty of being acknowledged accurately when the social world only sees and codes behaviour and appearance in binary terms. The authors recognised the heterogeneous relationships that can be had with the body, dysphoria, and with any potential process of transition.

M. Paz Galupo has done work on trans people's experiences of sexual orientation labels and identity (Galupo et al., 2016). This has more recently been followed, by Galupo and others, with attention paid to how microaffirmations (Galupo et al., 2018) or microaggressions (Pulice-Farrow et al., 2019) by romantic partners may affect gender non-conforming and agender people. Both articles report thematic analyses of small-scale survey data (n=161, 85 gender non-conforming, 76 agender). Affirmative themes highlighted multifaceted interplay with language and wider social interactions and participation. For example, validation could manifest not only through recognition and use of correct language and the avoidance of unwanted language, but correcting others and acknowledgement/active engagement regarding microaggressions and mistakes. The details of partner interactions (beyond simple professed support) may therefore have extensive ramifications for wider experiences of family, work and communities, or for resilience and confidence across any and all contexts.

It has been increasingly recognised that trans and gender diverse communities often occupy digital as well as (or even, rather than) physical spaces, with specific and important ramifications (Horak, 2014; Marciano, 2014; Nirta, 2017; Pearce, 2018). The ability of one to present oneself as non-binary in digital space has been recognised, particularly in the context of Facebook's gender options (Williams, 2014), yet Bivens (2017) has expulsed underlying design decisions as fundamentally embedding the gender binary into the construction of software. To contextualise further:

> Facebook's gender field type was originally programmed to accept more than two values: 1 = female, 2 = male, and 0 = undefined. While a zero is inadequate in many ways, it is still a value beyond the binary of ones and twos. From a user's perspective – looking only at the user interface, not the database – the only non-binary option was to leave the field blank. This coding practice grants validity to binary genders while erasing non-binary genders, but it also produces conditions that allow for existence outside of the binary. The material reality of three accepted values in the database transgresses a rigid binary, yet falls short of a fluid spectrum, positioning the database somewhere in-between. (Bivens, 2017: 884)

While this is suggestive of a liminal production of non-binary digital materiality, Bivens explains how by 2008, Facebook added a mandatory, binary gender field on sign-up. Users could no longer leave gender blank (whereby a user could be coded as 0/undefined), and so even if selecting a custom gender from 2014 onwards, 'deep in the database, users who select custom gender options are re-coded – without their knowledge – back into a binary/other classification system that is almost identical to the original 2004 database storage programming' (Bivens, 2017: 885). While self-determination has been made possible in a sense, it remains fundamentally illusory and superficial. The gender binary is protected and preserved in such a context by the capitalist motivation for gendered advertisement, and the industrial sense that a significant aspect of the value of personal data still rests in its ability to be gendered for such a purpose. A parallel may be drawn with healthcare, where non-binary possibilities are being explicitly proclaimed by providers. Yet simultaneously, how bodies are understood, and gender-affirming medical interventions provided, are fundamentally binarised as (broadly transmasculine or transfeminine) in both the socialisation and training of practitioners. Further, in work on recognising the importance of acknowledging non-binary youth in health research, Frohard-Dourlent et al. (2017: 7) highlight similar possibilities of superficiality in research, 'including gender identity questions in a study where there is no intention to engage in gender-based analysis creates the impression of inclusion, but ultimately erases non-binary peoples' [sic] presence in the research, wasting their time by invalidating their contribution'.

Nicholas (2018) argues that negative social responses towards non-binary gender diversity stems from 'binary genderism' in addition to transphobia, and the latter is insufficient as a conceptual frame for theorising negative social responses towards non-binary people and identities. They argue for specific shifts in professional practice through the queering of educational norms regarding how gender is understood and reinscribed. They highlight the production of allophilia – 'a positive feeling and attitude of openness toward an outgroup' (Alfieri and Marta, 2011: 99) – within various school-based initiatives in various countries. Yet the question of how to implement any holistic, paradigm-shifting reconceptualisation of gender as it pertains to healthcare providers or members of trans communities is complicated by first, a lack of voice among gender-diverse people articulating that there are problems in these settings, and second, potential resistance from (clinical or community) 'gender experts', who do not necessarily recognise there is anything for them to learn (or acknowledge) regarding any issue with the foundations of their conceptualisations of gender/sex.

Conclusion

This chapter has aimed to contextualise and orient the now-broad literatures on trans and gender-diverse identities and experiences. By presenting a critical history (or genealogy) of trans possibility, I hope to have supported the case that gender experiences that challenge and are challenged by a binary paradigm have been present for longer than intelligible identity categories. Gender-diverse communities and the structural provision of gender-affirming medical interventions have grown up together over the 20th century, accommodating and resisting each other as gender has been produced, performed or insisted in changing ways.

The development of an empirical sociology of trans experiences has had specific benefits. For example, Love (2014: 174, emphasis added) points out that 'accounting for *material* experience' positioned transgender studies as able to more effectively account for trans embodiment. Recognition of the explicit presence of participants not identifying as male or female in older research has attempted to demonstrate value in revisiting such work with the benefit of a contemporary lens. Second, this grounds such non-binary research within an existing research narrative.

Trans sociology has come a long way since it first explicitly emerged over twenty years ago, with continued engagement over issues including body image, embodiment, practices of care, identity formation and narrative, experiences of discrimination, and the impacts of these debates on communities and policies. However, as I have highlighted, empirical attention to the experiences and voices of non-binary people in particular has been limited, despite being increasingly acknowledged within theoretical discussions, and culturally visible.

Notes

[1] To quote the non-binary comedian Eddie Izzard, 'They're not women's clothes. They're my clothes. I bought them.' See: https://twitter.com/eddieizzard/status/ 519196883215192066?lang=en

[2] Best illustrated by Harold Garfinkel's account of 'Agnes' – a trans woman who, having stolen her mother's oestrogen from the age of 12, successfully convinced clinicians that she was intersex. Agnes only revealed this to her doctors, and Garfinkel himself, years after she had accessed the care she needed. For the full account and an excellent contextualising abstract, see Garfinkel (2006).

[3] A historical example would be Corbett v Corbett 1970, which annulled the marriage of April Ashley to Arthur Corbett on the basis that she was 'legally male'. A contemporary example would be the requirement to present 'medical evidence' in the form of two reports from medical practitioners or psychologists as part of being considered for a gender recognition certificate. This was first possible under the Gender Recognition Act 2004. Predictably, the 2004 Act does not recognise non-binary genders. A consultation on updating the Act took place in 2018 where the importance of non-binary recognition was emphasised in third-sector organisational responses. At the time of writing, the response from the Government Equalities Office has seen significant delay. Following a similar consultation, the Scottish Government decided not to recognise non-binary genders within legislation.

[4] Primary care practitioners still make referrals to, and have care duties transferred from GICs. Despite this, as well as the recommendation to provide bridging prescriptions due to lengthy waiting times, few primary care practitioners have detailed familiarity/confidence with trans healthcare, and there is no consistent or systematic training on the subject within UK university medical education.

[5] This term was used within anthropological literature to refer to a wide range of North American First Nation gender identities across different tribes. The term

is now understood as a slur, due to its origin from a French word for prostitute. The term *two-spirit* is now preferred as an umbrella term, originating from First Nation communities; however, tribally specific terms may be considered to offer the greatest respect and specificity (Epple, 1998).

6   Historically it was deemed necessary by medical practitioners that, in order to be socially accepted, trans people needed to hide their trans status, even relocating and establishing an entirely new social network when post-transition. This practice has been criticised as preventing the normalisation of trans narratives, as well as limiting trans communities and political mobilisation by creating pressure for self-erasure, even from each other (Namaste, 2000).

7   This term has been increasingly problematised due to positioning a 'cis appearance' as 'the' singular desired outcome, and implying that those who do not 'pass' have subsequently failed – which also reinforces Western beauty standards (with passing often related to attractiveness), disproportionately disadvantaging people of colour, and poor, fat and older people.

8   Enforced passing here means when trans/non-binary people allow or actively encourage others to position them as the gender they were assigned at birth (that is, pass themselves as cisgender) for work, comfort or safety reasons.

9   Gagné and Tewksbury's definition specifically differentiates between transsexual and transgender. Transgender in their context did not include people who sought medical transition, but otherwise included a wide range of gender diversity and non-conformity, including cross dressers and drag queens.

10   'Particularity' is defined as the quality of being individual, and thus a clinician's ability to respond to particularity will inform how transgender identities are articulated within clinical dialogues.

11   See also the special issues of *Transgender Studies Quarterly*: 'The Issue of Blackness' 4(2); 'Trans-in-Asia, Asia-in-Trans' 5(3); 'Trans Studies en las Américas' 6(2).

12   For more information, see: http://thefeministwire.com/2013/07/checking-our-privilege-working-together-notes-on-virtual-trans-communities-truscum-blogs-and-the-politics-of-transgender-health-care/

13   These 860 respondents did not include people who were living part time as one gender and part time as another, as might be the case with a binary-oriented trans person who may, for example, be out to friends but not family/work.

14   Important examples of this include the pervasive culture of religious conservatism that exists in certain parts of the US, which may result in serious fears of discrimination, rejection and ridicule. Also the private healthcare system of the US changes the dynamic and implications of receiving healthcare, with poorer individuals likely to avoid visiting a doctor if at all possible due to costs (whether uninsured or underinsured), or due to the risk of losing a job if taking time to attend medical appointments, which is far less possible under the legal framework of the UK.

15   The journal has since been renamed *International Journal of Transgender Health*.

2

Doing and being: my relationship with this work, and how it was done

> [I]t is necessary (for me, at least) to go beyond critical scholarship, which explains contradictions in the world, to activist scholarship, which attempts to resolve those contradictions, to bring about actual change. (Kobayashi, 2001: 55)

Introduction

Design and execution of this research were informed by minority group, insider politics (Zinn, 1979; Kanuha, 2000), emphasising the importance of ethical rigour and emancipatory political potential in its applications. This coalesced into an overarching set of ideas about how to approach research with trans/gender diverse communities (Vincent, 2018b). I begin this chapter with a detailed explanation of the research design. I then shift from the 'how' to the 'why', embedding my decisions in relation to the wider methods literature. My construction of mixed media diaries – which allowed diary keepers to record entries via any number of creative forms – is explained and justified, together with discussion of semi-structured interviews, and how the research was executed. I then discuss how the data was analysed. As non-binary narratives have limited precedent as a named category, the stories that the participants tell in relation to identity illustrate new possibilities of being. I draw on symbolic interactionism and social constructionism in order to conceptualise how social meaning is produced, which underpinned my reading of the data in the analytic process.

I then articulate how I addressed questions of recruitment, ethics and rapport, respectively. I then discuss what I believe to be an underemphasised aspect of research methods – my relationship with the work. This might be considered particularly salient because I began articulating a non-binary identity myself during the project (though only explicitly after data collection was completed). I would contend that this in and of itself is neither more nor less relevant than contexts where researchers have an unchanged gender identity throughout a given project (cis or trans), as such a critical reflection provides context with regard to researcher motivations and approaches. I then provide orienting demographic information about participants. The chapter closes with an acknowledgement of limitations.

Research design: data collection strategy and practicalities

The project used a multi-method, qualitative research design. Non-binary participants were invited to keep diaries. These were subsequently sent back to me for preliminary analysis. I then arranged follow-up interviews with participants through the summer and autumn of 2015. Interview data was transcribed, and analysed side-by-side with the diary material.

The diaries were kept by participants for four months, from the beginning of February to the end of May, 2015. This timeframe aimed to strike a balance between being long enough for the potentiality of community and/or medical happenings to occur, but without being so long as to unreasonably burden participants. The use of diary keeping over a four-month period is an example of an intensive, short-term, longitudinal method (Fraley and Hudson, 2014). This allows not only for frequent and ongoing reflection on lived experiences, but for participants to potentially revisit their diaries prior to their return in order to make amendments, or to produce entries inspired by their own earlier contributions. The function of the semi-structured interviews (to discuss diary contents and to collaboratively produce meanings with participants about experiences that had occurred during the diary keeping and also more generally) allowed for multiple levels of insight into participant experiences and perceptions. While the diaries in and of themselves emphasised freedom of direction and depth, the interviews complemented this through more targeted questioning, and the clarifying benefit of dialogue. The fixed length of time for the diary-keeping period positioned the research design as time-based (rather than event-based, whereby a certain minimum number of predefined occurrences are needed to trigger the end of data production), to allow participants definitive knowledge of the length of their participation (Iida et al., 2012). The emphasis on the depth of data, rather than quantity of infrequent events (potentially including GIC appointments, or other necessary medical care) so as to reduce the timeframe of fieldwork, also has the benefit of greater accessibility for those who experienced barriers to the ease of recording their diaries.

Each participant was posted an A5, 192-page, lined, hardback notebook to use during the project if they wished. It was made clear that use of the provided book was not compulsory. Articulating to participants that entries could instead be produced using other media, particularly on computers, was important to maximise the potential range of expression seen in the diaries. Each diary included three pages of guidance for participants to reference as needed. They contained open-ended advice on the topics for consideration, as well as a protocol for practicalities including naming any computer files, saving digital diary entries and how to return the diaries.

Diaries were posted to participants' addresses of choice, using a name specified for this purpose by each participant. This was an important factor to consider as name-use may be situational and conditional for trans/non-binary people, particularly if not out. Some participants used names for postage that differed from the name they wished to be referred by in all other communication.

Participants were encouraged to write (or otherwise produce entries) in their diaries as frequently as possible, without being made to feel pressured to 'produce data'. During recruitment, many of the participants asked how often they should use their diaries. This was indicative of a range of concerns, including whether they would have enough time to commit to the project, and anxiety over having 'enough' to say. I emphasised that there was no 'correct' way to use the diary, but also suggested that being able to include something every week would be desirable. I also recognised some people might prefer fewer, longer entries, while others might favour producing a larger number of smaller entries. I therefore needed to negotiate the tension between participants being given space to tell their stories in their own ways, while not being unclear – such that participants lacked direction or experienced uncertainty about what to do.

Engagement with diaries was encouraged by sending weekly 'reminder' emails to participants. The decision to do this was supported by work done by Horvath et al. (2007), who in their project received all diaries back on time except one (out of 26, which was only a day late) when sending daily email reminders. A previous study by Usdan et al. (2004) did not send email reminders, and had an 82 per cent non-completion rate. My experience was similar to Horvath et al. – all participants (who did not explicitly drop out at some earlier point) returned their diaries, with almost all on time.

The weekly emails also acted as a useful way to develop rapport with participants, many of whom would reply to these messages. I ensured that the content of the messages differed every week, in order to avoid essentially sending a repetitive and unengaging piece of spam mail. In the messages I would offer potential suggestions of how participants might approach their engagement with the project, and also provided links to online material concerning diaries, or queer content that I thought might be found interesting. Finn, for example, said of the emails 'They're really helping me structure some entries and know what's relevant to put in'. Alex responded to one weekly reminder that they felt 'A bit adrift' and that they 'just worry about putting stuff that isn't going to be of any use'. While this demonstrated Alex's commitment through their concern, it was also a useful chance to engage with them, and offer guidance and advice. Many of the participants used the weekly emails as a way to 'check in', offering their assurances that the diary had been received at the outset, and they were continuing to engage with the project. In order to allow time for organisation, I used the final month of the reminder emails to prompt arrangements for conducting an interview with each participant.

On completion of the diary-keeping period, participants returned their diaries using a pre-paid stamped addressed envelope (included when diaries were sent out). Those participants who made diary entries digitally returned their entries by email. In advance of the interviews, all participant diaries were read and used to produce a general interview protocol. Before each interview, additional questions were added which related to the specific content of the individual participant's diary – such as clarification or discussion of particular entries. Thus, guides were idiosyncratic yet maintained comparability. Interviews were conducted in different locations at the convenience and comfort of participants. Locations included private meeting rooms booked at the University of Leeds, the participant's home, or public spaces such as cafés. Participants assured their comfort with their interview location prior to initiation. In cases where it was not possible for a face-to-face meeting for the interview, video calls via Skype were used. Six out of the 18 interviews were conducted remotely.

The number of questions prepared for each interview also allowed for an approximation of how long interviews would take, which was useful for both researcher and participant (Turner, 2010). Interviews were estimated to take one hour, although most participants were both able and willing to continue beyond this (in cases where a participant needed to finish by a certain time, these times constraints were observed). Interview length ranged from 47 to 140 minutes, with an average length of 90 minutes. The extensive nature of these interviews was a result of the depth and breadth of the majority of the participants' answers, and the passion with which interviews were approached.

Mixed media diaries and semi-structured interviews

Participants were invited to express themselves freely during the period of diary keeping, and could articulate their thoughts and feelings using any media they preferred. Resultant data included hand-written and typed prose, audio recording, poetry, doodles, collages, photography and drawings. In addition to participant preference, the goal of this was to avoid inherently privileging any one mode of communication over another.

Using diary keeping as a research method provided a range of advantages. Alaszewski (2006: 33) points out how diaries 'provide a rich source of data for researchers who wish to explore the development of an individual life, and the activities and relationships of particular groups in society'. The research questions specifically ask how participants' gender identities are negotiated in relation to particular settings, justifying a method that allowed participants to record interactions *they* deemed relevant. Bolger et al. (2003: 580) point out how diaries allow 'the examination of reported events and experiences in their natural, spontaneous context', reducing the time between an experience occurring and it being recorded. Research methods such as interviews or focus groups in isolation are comparably disadvantaged, as greater retrospection is relied on for participant recall. Gaps and inaccuracies in recall of a longitudinal account are then considerably more likely.

Hyers et al. (2006) note in their discussion of using daily diaries to examine everyday prejudice-related experiences that retrospective methods (interviews or focus groups) tend to result in discussions of more extreme and unusual happenings due to their memorable nature. This potentially obscures more routine happenings and interactions, which are important sites of identity negotiation. Hyers et al. also mention how the discussions of particularly sensitive topics may mean 'that coping mechanisms, including efforts at sense making, may create distortions in recall' (2006: 317). The diary method encourages participants to create a record of their thoughts and feelings in relation to their gender identities soon after an interaction. Thus, one can gain access to a more intimate and detailed sense of the social phenomena under study. This is the case whether that interaction is with an institution or social structure, another person or within oneself – the cultural, interpersonal and intrapsychic[1], as respectively framed within a symbolic interactionist framework (Jackson and Scott, 2010).

Precedent for the use of diaries which go beyond text can be seen in the work of Bragg and Buckingham (2008), who used scrapbook-style diaries to conduct media research with young people. They followed up with interviews, focus groups and surveys, highlighting how diaries can synergise as part of a multi-method research design. When commenting on the outcomes of their research, Bragg and Buckingham (2008: 121) noted that the 'voices' that emerged from the scrapbooks could be very different when compared with how participants gave of themselves in the interview environment – 'some wrote extensively in their scrapbooks but were shy in interviews, and vice versa'. My hope was that combining methods which used different forms of expression would make self-expression more accessible – helping to access a wider range of voices, and thus richer data. The method allows for examination of patterns in the experiences and feelings of non-binary people, while recognising the power of individual voices. Flexibility with the diary medium also served to be emancipatory through the lens of disability, as multiple participants expressed that producing data with a computer helped mitigate the barriers of both dyslexia, and chronic fatigue syndrome.[2]

Finally, I suggest that the method is particularly appropriate for gender-diverse research. Plummer (2003: 522) has indicated how innovative methods such as 'drama, personal narrative with multiple voices, and poetry' have been used to improve access to marginalised voices. This destabilises hegemonic notions of 'correct form' within the research paradigm, opening up new possibilities. This can also be applied to interviewing practices (Kong et al., 2001).

Both the importance and extent of interview use within sociology are captured by Benney and Hughes' (1956: 137) claim that 'sociology has become the science of the interview'. The use of follow-up semi-structured interviews is highly compatible with diaries, as limitations encountered when using each method alone may be avoided, by filling each other's gaps. Bolger et al. (2003) note how the personality traits of participants (such as conscientiousness, or forgetfulness with diary-keeping) or health factors (such as cognitive impairments, or addiction) may create selective biases or omissions in diary data. In contrast, the environment of the interview means that data production is more structured, able to be observed directly, and 'guided' by the researcher to some extent. Further, while diaries allowed for detailed recall and reflection on events and experiences while relatively fresh in participants' minds, the opportunity to reflect on and discuss interactions at a later time in the interview setting allowed access to a different set of related data. Capturing a participant's impression of an experience at one time may be quite different from their impression later on, by which time introspection or further experiences may have shifted the personal meaning (or beliefs surrounding) the experience.

In order to minimise disruption when interviewing participants, I travelled to locations convenient and local to them wherever possible. In cases where there were restrictive travel costs and a lack of mutually possible meeting times, video interviews via Skype were used as a cost- and time-effective solution. Concerns over potentially significant differences between remote and in-person interviews have been raised (Irvine et al., 2013). Counter to this, it has been argued that synchronous (real-time) environments using video, while not identical to face-to-face interviewing, are significantly similar – particularly when the interview is unstructured or semi-structured (Sullivan, 2012). Ensuring a two-way video link in addition to audio meant that each person's body language and facial expression could be seen by both researcher and participant, allowing a closer approximation to interaction in person. While drawbacks have also been identified in using Skype interviews such as increased risk of withdrawal, or technological difficulties acting as a barrier to rapport (Deakin and Wakefield, 2014), many of these were ameliorated by earlier interactions with participants in relation to making interview arrangements, and during the diary phase of research. None of the participants who were interviewed withdrew from the study.

The interviews gave me the opportunity to ask participants about themes that emerged from the diaries collectively, and also to follow up on content related to an individual's diary contents specifically. This might have been to clarify the intended meaning of a diary passage or to explore my interpretations of their words, to reflect on any changes or developments since an entry, or to explore a particular issue in greater depth. Such questions intimately linked the diaries and the interviews, but some interview questions were also inspired by the main research questions without reference to the diary material. The resultant data was analysed collectively.

Multi-method epistemology and analytical strategy

Multi-method research poses particular challenges to analysis, given the different forms the data takes. I took inspiration from multiple frameworks – centrally, symbolic interactionism and a social constructionist approach – in order to synthesise a frame that could be applied with an appropriate degree of flexibility. Thematic analysis had the advantage of allowing disparate data types within diaries to be concurrently assessed. Tuckett (2005) has considered how thematic analysis of qualitative data works in practice, in relation to a symbolic interactionist framework. As symbolic interactionism recognises that the meaning ascribed to an object or idea can vary (Benzies and Allen, 2001), comparison between different participants was vital in suggesting explanations and recognising any social patterns.

Symbolic interactionism (SI) considers the meanings ascribed to objects and actions by social actors. Williams (2008: 849) points out how SI differed from most mid-20th century sociological practice, in that it did not make 'the epistemological assumption that the social sciences could be modelled after the biological and physical sciences to produce verifiable "facts" that explain social behaviour and predict future behaviour'. SI has a history of being anti-positivist and interpretive. Further, by drawing on SI, I reject the premise that microsociological knowledge can be acquired or generated independently from the 'subject'.

SI is rooted in the philosophical tradition of pragmatism. This system of thought holds that reality is understood in terms of the different perspectives that individuals may hold, rather than modelling a singular (objectively knowable) world. While an objective material world may exist, pragmatism recognises that all understanding of the world must pass through the lens of human experience, which is unavoidably constructed and constrained by social context (Hamati-Ataya, 2014). The absence of an objective truth about the world does not preclude the existence of the world, separate and apart from individuals. Rather, individuals act on the basis of the meaning that things have for them, and it is this interaction between individual and object that produces meaning (Benzies and Allen, 2001). Individuals form their views and construct their own truths of the world, on the basis of the interactions they experience – with other people, objects and ideas. The role of (social) scientific enquiry thus becomes 'a moral endeavour', concerned not with an abstract knowledge production for its own sake, but with the purpose of application to the improvement of human lives (Williams, 2008: 850). Thus, my theoretical position may be understood as ontologically relativistic – the purported understandings of reality are not attempting to access any objective truth, but all have value in and of themselves, derived through *application*.

During the development of SI, two separate branches of pragmatism were used – by Mead (1934) on the one hand, and Dewey (1905) on the other. Lewis and Smith (1980) argue that Mead's pragmatism has been conceived as philosophical realism, which has macrosociological overtones. In contrast, Dewey produced a 'nominalist' pragmatism

– which recognises macrosocial structures, but attributes greater importance to individual interactions in shaping identities and behaviours (Lewis and Smith, 1980). The use and understanding of SI in this work leans towards Dewey's position, with a focus on how the meanings that objects have for individuals are personal, subjective and symbolically associated with objects however the actor interprets them (Ritzer, 2008).

Qualitative methods are most often chosen when using SI, due to their usefulness in elucidating nuanced analysis from microsociological interactions. Using diaries as a method creates a shift from 'participant observation towards the observation of participation' (Tedlock, 1991: 69). Tedlock describes how this change also alters the research dynamic away from a researcher-self versus researched-other to a 'single narrative ethnography'. This allows for co-production of knowledge between participants and investigator, fitting with the epistemological premise within SI that 'rejects the idea of a disembodied researcher' (Williams, 2008: 849). Further, this assists in avoiding a problematic power dynamic that can be seen particularly in historical medical research on, rather than with, trans people.

I wish to provide some additional clarification about how I relate SI to a broader social constructionist approach. I draw particularly from Gary Alan Fine's (1993) work that argues social constructionism is one of six areas of empirical social scientific work where SI has made significant contributions (along with social coordination theory, the sociology of emotions, self and identity theory, macro-interactionism and policy-oriented research). Fine notes that as interactionism 'fractured' from roughly the 1960s onwards as different scholars taught increasingly divergent versions of the framework, while broadly holding to core concepts originating with Herbert Blumer (1969) – 'that we know things by their meanings, that meanings are created through social interaction, and that meanings change through interaction' (Fine, 1993: 64). Further, the pragmatic basis for SI should, it follows, embrace innovation in seeking to develop conceptual tools optimised for purpose – avoiding a 'fortress mentality' (Fine, 1993: 66). It is fitting that Fine frames the social constructionist approach as permitting 'interactionists to examine dynamic, historical processes affecting the social system, such as the medicalization of deviance' (1993: 75), given the historic relationship between gender diversity and medical intervention. Others have considered the relationship between constructionism and SI in sub-disciplinary specific contexts (for example, Leeds-Hurwitz, 2006). I argue that even where specific reference to gender is made, as Leeds-Hurwitz (2006: 237) does in arguing that social constructionism is 'particularly appropriate to examine the socialization to gender that occurs within the family', this does not especially engage with gender as gender *identity*, and how its conceptualisation and expression can be understood as navigated/ negotiated through interaction. Leeds-Hurwitz makes a particularly bold distinction between SI and social constructionism as essentially micro- and macro- driven, stating 'symbolic interactionism emphasizes making sense of self and social roles, whereas social constructionism focuses more broadly on making sense of the nature and structure of the social world' (Leeds-Hurwitz, 2006: 238). I contend that Fine (1993) offers a more nuanced reading of the relationship between frameworks by considering how interactionists (and by implication, constructionists) may be widely situated across a range of debates – particularly naming 'micro/macro', 'agency/structure', and 'realist/ interpretivist'. Like gender, it's fair to argue these are false binaries, with the possibility of being understood as spectra or spaces within which one is situated – or moves.

SI is epistemologically well suited to the study of gender, and has previously been rehabilitated in order to act as a framework for a feminist sociology of sexuality (Jackson and Scott, 2010). In arguing that interactionism accounts for the processes by which sexuality is constituted through cultural, interpersonal and intrapsychic interactions, the same approach can be adapted for an analysis of (non-binary) gender identities. Indeed, Harrison et al. (2012: 20) specifically state that this awaits further study when asking 'how does nuance or multiplicity in gender identity and expression play out when interacting with gender policing structures and forces?' Space constraints necessitate sidestepping potentially lengthy engagement with debates about relativism and the conceptualisation of identity within sociology. I simply mean to use the basic scaffolding of SI to make sense of an empirical engagement with the situated, ongoing evolution of gender identity, as reported/performed by individuals who related themselves to constructed, personal articulations of non-binary.

An iterative analytic process was used, in that the multi-method nature of the research meant coding and analysis began before all data was collected. In the first instance, this began by reading participant diaries as they were returned. The nature of researching non-binary gender identities justified a combination of inductive and deductive coding, which has sociological precedent (Fereday and Muir-Cochrane, 2006). Inductive coding, where codes are generated without predeterminations, was necessary because of the lack of attention that non-binary identities had received at the time of the research. However, the small amount of specific research that exists (Harrison et al., 2012; Yeadon-Lee, 2016; Bolton, 2019), together with an anecdotal sense from community interaction and involvement meant that some deduction (and thus, deductive coding, informed by prior contexts) could be applied – particularly in relation to medical practice where some experiences are comparable to binary-oriented trans narratives (Burgwal et al., 2019).

No notes were made during the first read-through of each diary. This was in order to allow me to focus on the narrative sense of the data as a whole, and become closer to the raw data (Sandelowski, 1995). On a second read-through, initial themes were identified and colour coded, and cross-referenced with the other diaries. Themes were identified between diaries through cross-sectional comparison, and within diaries, between different entries over time (Thomson and Holland, 2003). Thematic interpretation of images, poetry and so on was frequently discussed during interviews, which allowed both an additional perspective and assessment of participant intentions. Regular academic supervision meetings also allowed for refinement of data analysis.

These read-throughs informed the construction of personalised topic guides. Each participant's topic guide contained core questions, but also notes of topics to discuss that were particular to individuals. For example, Finn included a poem in their diary but highlighted that much of the meaning was dependent on performance, therefore in the interview setting I asked Finn to read/perform the poem which lead to a discussion about it.[3] Recurring themes that were identified between diaries – for example, 'feeling insecure as trans' – inspired the wording of questions. There is a certain parallel with a grounded theory approach here (Glaser and Strauss, 1999) in that no assumptions were made about what would be found in the diaries, and by allowing diary content to inform interview guides, participant voices do not test existing theory, but rather produce it.

Following the participant interviews, the audio recordings were transcribed. This was done near-verbatim, with the only omissions being occasional conversational asides that did not pertain to the research (but within the interview setting, contributed to rapport). The same approach was then taken to the transcripts as to the diaries – an initial read-through without notes, followed by note making and coding that was then cross-referenced. Each interview was also compared with the participant's diary, and more broadly across the entire data set.

Recruitment

Emmel has highlighted how consideration of sample size practicality is given relatively little attention, and that 'to ask how big the sample size is or how many interviews are enough is to pose the wrong question. It is far more useful to show the ways in which the working and reworking of relationships between ideas and evidence in the research are a foundation for the claims made from that research' (Emmel, 2013: 137). This relates strongly to the notion of theoretical saturation – that is, the point at which it is believed that an increase in the sample size will not generate significant new codes or points of theoretical import (Guest et al., 2006). This concept is rooted in the context of work utilising grounded theory, and thus does not consider the additional dimension of a multi-method approach. However, the concept can still inform sample size decision making, by giving a sense of the ratio of labour to yielded themes.

Guest et al. (2006) conducted 60 interviews, coding and analysing in batches of six, so that originality of contribution and redundancy could both be looked at, in terms of the individual codes and their relative importance. While there is a precedent (arguably arbitrary and under-evidenced) for sample sizes of 30 participants within graduate and postdoctoral qualitative projects (Mason, 2010), Guest et al. found the yield of theoretically significant codes dropping off as early as following 12 interviews. With this evidence borne in mind, a sample size of 25 participants was originally decided. Given the large time investment required by participants, this number was chosen to allow for enough data to still be produced should several participants choose to withdraw, fail to submit diary entries, or if multiple participants only produce a very limited number of entries.

With hindsight this was a prudent decision, as seven participants withdrew from the project at various stages, leaving the final sample of 18 participants. This was for a range of reasons, including feeling unable to dedicate enough time to the project, personal reasons, and in one case, loss of the diary and unwillingness to perform a stand-alone interview. One participant, Jess, also lost her diary, but was willing to be interviewed for the project. Thus, 17 diaries and 18 interviews comprised the final data set.

In order to recruit participants, I produced a poster for use in both physical and digital spaces. To simplify the poster, the only criterion for participation mentioned was 'identifying outside of the gender binary', with the intention to explain further details and requirements on expression of interest. The poster also explained briefly what participants would be asked to do, and provided contact details, and a reference number to prove the ethical approval of the work by the University of Leeds. I also produced an information sheet, which was provided to any potential participants who made enquiries about the project. The information sheet spanned two A4 pages (in the original format), so as to avoid inundating potential participants with too much information. I included an explanation of what the project was investigating and why, along with full eligibility criteria, what was being asked of participants, and a description of participant rights, including withdrawal and anonymity. In order to recruit from communities, I produced a template email to be sent to online groups to request circulation of my poster within their membership. These documents were all ethically reviewed and found to be satisfactory by the University of Leeds Research Ethics Committee.[4]

Recruitment of participants was pursued through multiple avenues. These included networking at queer-oriented activist and academic events. In addition, I made contact with non-binary groups and spaces, both physically and digitally. Building on this, snowball sampling from individuals accessed in these ways allowed further access to non-binary members of LGBTQ communities and friendship networks (Atkinson and Flint, 2001). Calls for participation were also spread through digital networks such as Facebook, Tumblr and Twitter, with requests made for people to share the information widely.

A potential limitation of snowball sampling is that members of friendship networks are more likely to share experiences and beliefs, risking greater homogeneity when representing the population under consideration (Biernacki and Waldorf, 1981). It must be remembered that no piece of population research can claim to be 'truly' or 'completely' representative. I draw on Haraway's (1988) feminist concept of situated knowledges, in that knowledge generated is not positioned as generalisable 'fact', but can be used to inform theorisation – in this case, processes of identity negotiation. The synergy of the recruitment methods I used provided a sample with some cross-demographic variation, when considering that the number of people articulating a non-binary identity is relatively small in comparison to cisgender men and women. Estimating the size of the non-binary population is extremely difficult due to lack of reliable data and lack of cultural intelligibility, as well as shifting definitions of categorisation. However, detailed community-oriented work has estimated the non-binary population as up to 0.4 per cent (Titman, 2014). The reachable population for research will be significantly smaller.

Three specific non-binary-oriented groups were approached, with requests to distribute information about the project to their membership.

These were Non-Binary South West, the Non-Binary Inclusion Project, and the UK Non-Binary/GQ meet-up network (which exists specifically as a closed Facebook group, but which I was able to access with the assistance of existing members). The project was also posted on the 'Beyond the Binary' working group Facebook page. My recruitment poster was also displayed in the CliniQ waiting room in London, then the only UK sexual health service aimed specifically for trans people.

Posting on social media was an effective method of recruitment, with friends and community members reposting information to give a wider pool of potential interest. Digital recruitment methods did however highlight the importance of appreciating the loss of control the researcher experiences over whereabouts a call for participants may be shared. This was brought to my attention when I received multiple enquiries by email from interested persons in the US, despite my project recruiting from people living in the UK only. The inclusion of this criterion was in order to make the broad cultural context of the research more consistent and comparable across the sample.

Ethical considerations

Within a paradigm of working with participants rather than 'studying subjects', I considered it a reasonable ethical decision to give participants the choice of whether to be identifiable or not. The ethical consideration of that decision has been academically explored (Giordano et al., 2007). By assuming the state of anonymity to be essential, researchers risk 'acting paternalistically and might be denying participants' autonomy ... and/or depriving participants of a "voice" that confers personal meaning to their enjoinment to the research and its effect(s), outcomes, and goals' (Giordano et al., 2007: 265).

I do not claim that allowing participants to share their names is always ethically justifiable. Rather, this is a context-dependent decision that must be critically considered in relation to risk. The work only used first names, and I had no reason to doubt or question the ability of participants to accurately assess the meanings or impacts that real first-name use could have for them. Participants were also given the option to choose their pseudonym, if anonymity was preferred. Of the 18 participants, eight chose anonymity and ten chose to use their first name, demonstrating a slim majority of participants felt comfortable being identifiable. Several participants were glad to choose their own pseudonyms as it allowed them expression though the choice of a name they liked, or which held some personal significance. When participants chose to be anonymous and did not choose their pseudonym, I notified them of the pseudonym I gave them, so that they could identify themselves in the work more easily if they wanted to, once the thesis was made available. An interesting detail was that multiple participants felt able to use their name *as* their pseudonym, due to the name they identified with being chosen by themselves, and different from that given to them at birth. In some cases (such as Pig), this chosen name would not only be unrecognisable to anyone from whom anonymity would be desirable, but would also be recognisable to those who knew them in queer communities (whom they did not feel a need to be anonymised from, or may desire to be visible to). Names could thus disrupt the 'anonymised/identifiable' binary, through their intelligibility in some contexts, but not in others.

A range of safeguards were used to protect participants from potential harm. All participants signed a consent form before participation. This explicitly stated that participants were not required to share anything (in written/artistic form in the diaries, or verbally in the interviews) which they did not feel comfortable with. I outlined the right to withdraw from the project, with a specific deadline of one month following the date of the interview. Justification of this deadline was that proximity to the final submission of the PhD thesis risked the project if too little data remained without time for replacements to be found. However, no participants withdrew consent following their interview. Participants could also change their anonymity status (becoming anonymous when formerly identifiable, or vice versa) up to three months following their interview. The difference in dates reflected the comparative ease in anonymising/de-anonymising a participant relative to complete removal and replacement of an individual in the research.

Each method used had specific ethical considerations. As the diaries contained information on participants' gender identities (a personal and potentially sensitive topic), I advised participants to be mindful of when and where they wrote, and how they stored their diaries. In the case of handwritten diaries, participants were advised to keep them in a safe and secure location. For entries written or produced on a computer, I advised that files were stored in a well-hidden folder, or password protected to ensure privacy, where necessary. These precautions were particularly salient for participants who were not necessarily out regarding their gender identity. On receiving diaries, digital material was password protected, and physical material was kept in a locked filing cabinet, together with the signed consent forms.

Interviews also followed practices of sensitivity to ensure participant comfort during discussions. The negotiation of a non-binary identity is likely to be experienced as a sensitive topic, due to participants potentially having experience of stigma, discrimination or other upsetting associations in relation to their status (Lee, 1993). All but one participant described themselves as trans, therefore these minority stress factors are highly entwined with transphobia and cisgenderism (Kennedy, 2013). Before each interview began it was clearly communicated to each participant that they did not have to answer anything they were not comfortable with, and they did not have to give any reason for doing so. Further, they could end the interview at any time, without communicating a reason. Participants had the right to refuse consent for particular topics of conversation to be written about, without necessarily fully withdrawing from the project. These explicitly communicated concerns for participant wellbeing served to reassure participants and add to rapport building.

Building rapport

Schuman (1982: 22–3) draws attention to the importance of language in the research encounter, in saying 'all answers depend upon the way a question is formulated. Language is not a clean logical tool like mathematics that we can use with precision … as if this complexity were not enough, our answers are also influenced by who asked the question'. Given my extensive contact with participants prior to interview (via email), the development of rapport over time was important for interview success. Rapport was developed during the recruitment and diary-keeping phases by engaging with participants with respect and reciprocity, which synergises with feminist ethical practices (Oakley, 1981). Where asked, I shared my personal experiences and motivations with participants. Due to the interviews being undertaken after the diary-keeping period, some important interaction with participants had already occurred when participants enquired about participation, and via email in the form of the weekly email prompts. During recruitment for example, Leon wished to ask me a range of questions, to inform their decision about participating:

> Before I go any further, though, I wonder if you could let me know a bit more about yourself. What brought you to this research? What do you hope to achieve and what impact do you hope your research will have? How did you come to your research methods and what challenges do you envisage this particular methodology posing? What ideas/

theories/scholars/writers (academic and non-academic) have inspired you? (Leon, 34, email)

Answering Leon's questions in detail served to reassure them that my work was sympathetic towards non-binary emancipatory politics, rather than critical or transphobic, as with some scholarship that has come before (Raymond, 1979; Jeffreys, 2014). My willingness to answer questions and discuss what brought me to a study of non-binary lives, and the political convictions which guide my approach, served to improve both my access to (and interactions with) participants.

It was important to continue to build a sense of trust and rapport with participants during the interviews. This was partly fostered through beginning the interaction by thanking the participant for their time and effort with the diary, and to affirm the pronoun(s) they wished to be used. While referring to the participant in the third person generally did not come up in the interview context, it was later important for accurate writing about participants. Further, this demonstrated to participants the centrality of their validity and respect in this research.

Where am I in this? Reflexive positioning and autoethnographic reflections

Having been defined as the 'thoughtful, self-aware analysis of the intersubjective dynamics between researcher and the researched' (Finlay and Gough, 2003: ix), reflexivity offers important ways to perform social scientific research with heightened ethical considerations (Wasserfall, 1993). The demand for greater (and sometimes difficult) reflection from the researcher is an attempt to sensitively address power relations between researchers and their subjects/collaborators (England, 1994) – particularly where participants are already members of a disenfranchised population, as is the case for the non-binary people in this research.

Audrey Kobayashi (2001) has discussed the negotiation of the personal and the political in critical qualitative research in the context of her, as a researcher, introspecting on the wellbeing of her participants. Valuably, Kobayashi underscores the importance of both understanding and taking responsibility for how one may set in motion complex emotions, which 'flow back and forth' in the course of a research encounter. While this may be more obvious in the context of an interview and how respondents may feel about personal questions concerning identity, diary keeping also entailed a potential impact. Such considerations shaped the ethical dimensions of my methodology.

It has been argued that while 'being reflexive' is often recognised as important in social scientific research, but the practicalities of 'doing reflexivity' have not been emphasised (Mauthner and Doucet, 2003). Scholars can still problematically infer that 'the researcher, the method and the data are separate entities rather than reflexively interdependent and interconnected' (Mauthner and Doucet, 2003: 414). With this in mind, my personal relationship with this project is significant, and I believe benefits from contextualisation. While this work is not primarily autoethnographic, my history and identity have influenced important dimensions such as participant access and interactions.

My experiences of trans narratives have been highly personal and poignant. During 2011–12 I was in a long-term relationship with a trans man, during which time I was indirectly exposed to some of the emotional and bureaucratic difficulties of accessing gender-affirming medical interventions through the NHS. These were illustrative of the potential for systemic road blocks to progression, or unequal treatment between cis and trans patients. In addition, I mourned the suicide of a close trans friend, who had not only struggled with accessing medical services but also with unrelated mental health conditions, all of which was compounded by transphobic stigma. Such personal exposure to the tremendous difficulties that trans people can experience, and the deficiencies in the systems that are designed to provide support, drives an activist dimension to my work in that the production of social change is as vital as the production of knowledge (Ackerly and True, 2010; Warner, 2013).

My PhD, which began in September 2013, was fundamentally driven by the aforementioned earlier experiences, and I had originally intended to look at the impacts of medical policy via the NHS on transmasculine transitions. I conceived this as being non-binary-inclusive, but it was only during the assessment process at the end of my first year of study that I was advised shifting to focus on non-binary gender identities would have a greater original claim.[5] Throughout this time, I explicitly conceived of myself as a cisgender researcher engaging with trans communities, and was cognisant of the tensions this could potentially produce (Tagonist, 2009). I continued to situate myself as cis for a long time out of caution, not wishing to 'inappropriately' overreach and claim something that I felt some affinity towards, but which might not be 'mine', or that I was something I might not 'be'. I wrote a couple of blog posts exploring this (between late 2015 and early 2016),[6] which contained some intriguing juxtapositions. I wrote that I did not experience any gender dysphoria (the 'truth' of which is difficult to answer – what constitutes dysphoria?), but that I had never liked, identified with, or felt comfortable with the concept of 'being a man'. I wrote of liminality – inspired by the contents of one participant's diary (Finn's), and the nucleation of material that forms parts of Chapter 4 of this book. I felt a great uncertainty – which gave way to anxiety – about how to situate myself, and why I might situate myself within a given identity. I have felt similarly about the concept of love – highly personal, ultimately impossible to 'verify' whether you *are* feeling it, but with a cultural hegemony that suggests 'when you find it, you will know'.

Ultimately, I have found it empowering to conceptualise my non-binary identity as at least partially my own choice – not a novel concept (Whisman, 1996), yet still politically inflammatory in many contexts. I have been forced to confront the question 'what makes *me* non-binary?', not so much because of any specific community pressure to justify myself but a deep internal insecurity that I may be, on some unconscious level, attempting to validate myself and my work politically as being 'from the community'. This was an insidious fear, and I ultimately believe, the wrong question to ask. Because I was really asking myself 'how do I know if I'm *really* non-binary?', suggesting an essential 'truth' to gender identity, independent of experience or agency. It was the fear I wasn't enough – the driving theme of the next chapter.

What is it that means I choose to articulate myself as non-binary, rather than as a gender non-conforming man, perhaps echoing Stoltenberg (2005)? The difference is, for me – at least at this time – political. I have chosen a category that feels preferable, and I have worked to make my home and bed within it. I believe there is enormous emancipatory potential in queer allegiance between people with different forms and experiences of gendered difference. Part of my fear was also that perhaps I was seeking to escape the uncomfortable reality that my assignment at birth (and associations that come from appearance, such that I am socially rendered fairly consistently as 'a man') affords me various undeserved and unjust privileges. I answer this essentially by saying that being sensitive to the ways in which one is privileged is not mutually exclusive with any particular gendered subjectivity. Further theorisation of male privilege is ripe for development, as Kortney Ziegler (2018) highlights in his piece 'The peculiarity of black trans male privilege': 'Although I'm less likely to be sexually assaulted because of the way I present my gender, this privilege is in exchange for becoming a visible target of racist practices designed to police young black manhood.' I do not draw any equivalence, but rather suggest that 'male' (and 'female') contain within them multiple axes for having advantage/disadvantage, legitimacy/ illegitimacy, safety/vulnerability, fit/misfit. When we talk about a person as being male or female, we are not isolating a single aspect of their being, but obscuring the relationships between many. I can engage with discussions of gendered privilege that might interrogate my socialisation, my mannerisms, my voice, my stature and so on, without being flattened to a single deficient category.

I do not conceive of my non-male identity as something that I 'discovered', or as something I necessarily 'always was', but rather as something that emerged out of emotional and introspective work. My sense of unease at challenging politically dominant trans ontologies reminded me of Talia Bettcher's (2014) article 'Trapped in the wrong theory: rethinking trans oppression and resistance'. Here she critiques the 'wrong-body model', as well as any notion that trans people *should* be rejecting any identity based in the gender binary on the basis that gender is an oppressive social construct. Her point is echoed by Bolton's summary of Foucault critiquing the notion of confessing an 'internal truth': 'rather than being released in the process of confession, one becomes subjected to regulatory power' (Bolton, 2019: 27). I am resistant to proclaiming my identity as internal truth, yet I am still regulated because the 'small print' detail of my self-concept is not able to be articulated if and when I say 'I'm non-binary'. I am regulated by unintelligibility, such that whether I let others assume I'm male or not varies with context (and correspondingly with anxiety about how I may be responded to, and how much energy I have for any discussion). If I don't allow the assumption, I must then consider how to communicate and account for myself. The confession raises questions from others (about what I want to do with my body, how I know, what this means), and the answers must be intelligible – even if one doesn't know, one is assumed to either want to 'transition' or not, and for that to *follow from* identity. My point is, that to navigate being 'out' as non-binary has demanded exceptional consideration about how to navigate this. It is not a choice made lightly, but can correspondingly be a source of validation – I am real because of the social and internal processes that have rendered me. I am also regulated by trans and gender-diverse communities, not only through the anxiety of being judged as invalid by someone, but also the fear that trying to articulate a relationship with gender that is in tension with the 'born this way' narrative may be politically weaponised.

Why are arguments for the ontological validity of identities that are based in biological work (that is, 'born this way' conceptualisations) afforded greater respectability than those based in sociological or philosophical perspectives? Because discourses are subject to an epistemological hierarchy. While it is easier to convince legislators and a general public of the necessity for legal protections – and to position bigotry as callous – with an essentialised explanation (be it for gender identity or sexuality), this strategic essentialism (Spivak, 1985) fails to challenge the inferior status held by minority groups. For example, if being gay or trans is acceptable *because* one is born that way, does that imply that if one were *not* born that way, it would no longer be acceptable? If we recognise a phenomenon – such as non-binary gender identities – as an acceptable thing to be, then causation ceases to matter. Aetiological research is controversial and inflammatory in the context of gender diversity due to the potential for a eugenics-oriented logic that may propose the ability to screen or test for trans status. This could be inspired by a drive to 'validate' diagnoses through a gatekeeping model of healthcare access, or to allow for prenatal screening and targeted termination. There is no motive to 'fix' or 'prevent from happening' that which is not viewed as broken.

It is also important to unpack the notion of 'choice' – my non-binary identity-as-choice is not equivalent to the choice of a meal, or an outfit. This is a false equivalency made to delegitimise political queerness through equalising it with viewing gender and sexual orientation as 'lifestyle'. Rather, my choice is the sharp end of the navigation of life; this reflection could be explored in much greater detail. These passages are somewhat confessional as well as exploratory – in being so, they draw attention to how difference tends to be encouraged to explain itself first. Are there any books about gender-diverse experience where a cisgender author dedicates space to a vulnerable reflection on their gendered subjectivity?[7]

I have critically interrogated my gendered subjectivity for years. I do not believe this gives me any kind of ontological superiority – I am no more or less valid than those who have not, or who have done so for longer. In such a context 'validity' is shorthand for 'worthy of acknowledgement and respect', which can be more readily afforded to white, middle-class academics who can use their access to education and sociolinguistic stylings to cultivate a politics of respectability. Or to put it another way – I'm not more real because of how I'm expressing this. Ultimately, I do not subscribe to a philosophical paradigm that sees value in attempting to 'test' whether non-binary identities are 'real' or not. Rather, I contend that non-binary identities are *meaningful* because of the social interactions they produce – within an individual, between different people, or with wider social structures or discourses.

Participant demographic information

Names followed by no asterisks are not anonymised. Those followed by one asterisk are pseudonyms chosen by me, and those followed by two asterisks are pseudonyms chosen by the participant specifically. The brackets after the name indicate the participant's pronoun(s). As identity and expression may change over time, it is important to recognise this information as situated, and from 2015. I am especially mindful that pronoun use may possibly have changed, particularly for any participant who may have renegotiated a binary-oriented identity[8] (discussed further in Chapter 4).

Alex (they, he): A white Welsh 20-year-old university student, living in South Yorkshire/Leeds. They identified as queer. They were polyamorous, and in an open relationship.

Ash (they): A white 33-year-old sex worker who lived in Northamptonshire. They identified as having a fluid sexuality, and were in a relationship.

Bobby★ (they): A white British 23-year-old student who lived in Surrey. They identified as pansexual, and were single.

Charlie (they): A white British 21-year-old student who lived in Nottingham. They identified as queer, and were in a relationship.

David★ (they): A white 31-year-old policy researcher who lived in London. They identified as gay, and were married.

Finn (they): A white British 22-year-old student who lived in Sheffield/Leeds. They identified as queer, and were in polyamorous relationships.

Frankie (they): A white British 25-year-old sexual health and wellbeing worker who lived in London. They identified as a queer dyke, and were in polyamorous relationships.

Hal★ (they): A white 42-year-old market researcher who lived in London. They were primarily attracted to men, and they were single.

Jamie★ (they): A white 24-year-old PhD student who lived in York. They identified as gay, and they were married.

Jen (she): A white Scottish 29-year-old PhD student who lived in Leeds. She identified as queer, and was in an open relationship.

Jess (she, they[9]): A white 26-year-old PhD student, teaching assistant and proof-reader, who lived in Manchester. She identified as pansexual (though tended not to define). Their relationship status was "complicated".

Leon★★ (they): A white 34-year-old lecturer, who lived in Nottingham. They identified as queer, and were in a civil partnership.

Mark (he): A white British 43-year-old personal carer who lived in Norwich. He identified as "mostly gay", and was "single-ish".

Pig (they, it): A white 30-year-old youth worker who lived in Manchester. They identified as queer, and had a long-term partner.

Rachel★★ (they): A white German Jewish 28-year-old student who lived in Manchester. They identified as a lesbian and were in a relationship.

Ricky★★ (they): A white British 43-year-old counsellor and trainer, who lived in Nottingham. They identified as bisexual, and they were married.

V★★ (he): A white British 28-year-old artist, writer, and performer who lived in Nottinghamshire. They described their sexuality as unfussed, and they were single.

Zesty (they, any): A mixed-race 22-year-old student chef who lived in Cairo/Leeds. They identified as polysexual, and they were single.

Participants lived in a total of 12 different cities or regions. Counties were used in cases where individuals lived in a location smaller than a city, in order to protect location privacy where necessary. The age range represented was 20–43 years, with an average of 29.1, and a median of 28. Ages were recorded at the point of recruitment to the project. Research by Harrison et al. (2012) suggested that (in a North American cultural context, at least) non-binary people were significantly less likely to be over the age of 45. An explanation of this may be due to the way language use has changed with relation to trans and gender-diverse people over the past several decades. This is similar to how 'transgender' has increasingly replaced the older term 'transsexual', both within academic literature and as an identity label (Stryker, 2008a). The specific 'naming' of non-binary/genderqueer people is recent in Western contexts. As Plummer (1995) put it, shifts in language have only recently allowed such stories to be told. Older people may be less likely to associate with labels which were not known or not used for much of their lives, yet the emergence of terms *can* allow for personal sense making and reconceptualisation at any age. The sample size of this project cannot be taken to be 'representative'; the experiences of older non-binary people remain an under-researched and valuable area for further study. Scholars should be mindful of the exclusion and flattening that happens when 'non-binary people' are assumed to be young – and similarly, thin, white, androgynous or 'alternative' in style.

The above demographic data was collected in order to further contextualise the reached community members in this research.

All participants except one identified their ethnicity as white. This runs contrary to Harrison et al.'s (2012) non-binary population data, where 30 per cent were non-white, but in a North American context. While the 2011 UK census data estimates the proportion of the UK population who identify themselves as white at 81.9 per cent, lack of racial/ethnic diversity may be symptomatic of snowball sampling. Alternatively, compounding minority statuses (non-binary, non-white) may result in more vulnerable/marginalised individuals who are more difficult to access (Mutch et al., 2013). Educational attainment was significantly higher than the general population, with all participants except Ash (who had completed A-levels) currently undertaking, or having already attained, at least one degree. This may be indicative of the class positions of participants; however more detailed consideration of class intersection was not undertaken. A wide range of different descriptors of sexuality were given. This is perhaps to be expected, as non-binary gender identities disrupt the binary foundation on which sexuality categories such as gay and straight are based. Despite this, some participants did identify as gay or lesbian – though no participants identified as straight/heterosexual. It is also noteworthy that the majority of participants had prior experience of diary keeping. It is possible that advertisement of the method in recruitment material had an impact on the interest in participation, such that individuals with a lack of writing experience may have been put off prior to initial enquiry. This may be positioned as a limitation of the research; however, the method may have also served to make the research more attractive to some respondents.

Limitations of methods and recruitment

It is important to recognise potential limitations of using diaries and interviews as research methods. The length of time and level of commitment required from participants in keeping a diary was significant. This placed a relatively heavy burden on individuals, and contributed to the high dropout rate (of seven, from an original 25). This is common in diary-based research (Bolger et al., 2003; Schroder et al., 2003), though I attempted to reduce withdrawal by clearly highlighting the nature of the commitment before participation was confirmed, together with the use of weekly reminder emails. Participant autonomy is, however, privileged within the diary-keeping method because, as Ruth Holliday highlights with the use of video diaries, participants may go back to consider earlier entries and edit as they see fit before passing their entries to the researcher. Holliday

(2000: 510) posits that this sort of research method therefore offers participants the 'potential for a greater degree of reflexivity', which may increase participants' confidence in the accuracy of their data in reflecting their views and experiences. As with other research methods, participants may attempt to adapt their tone and answers to fulfil perceived expectations of the researcher. I attempted to minimise this by clearly signposting the freedom of expression participants had in producing entries relating to their sense of negotiating their gender identities. Interviews may be accused of focusing on exceptional, 'more than everyday' events; however, this was ameliorated by the multi-method approach.

The sample itself can also be critiqued, in that more intersections of diversity may have been possible through a more nuanced recruitment strategy. Although the question was not asked specifically when collecting demographic information, many participants in their diaries and interviews made specific reference to experiences of disability. Thus, intersections between non-binary gender identity and disability were able to be explored, while race (for example) was not. The theory of situated knowledges (Haraway, 1988) challenges any claim that individual representation of a particular marginalisation (disability, race, class status, age, sexuality and so on) grants group representation in and of itself.

While not a 'limitation' per se, research is certainly affected by a researcher's personal relationship with a research population. Whether or not the researcher has lived experience will affect (and shape) the knowledge produced (Griffith, 1998). Despite identifying as queer prior to conducting this research, I positioned myself as an outsider researcher due to my not (then) identifying explicitly as non-binary. The process of conducting the research significantly shaped my relationship with my own gender, and this was certainly informed by the manner in which participants responded to me. For example, within interview settings, informal aspects of conversation (not recorded) could involve participants articulating thoughts expressly about *our* community, rather than *their* community. Despite my ambiguities regarding identity labels, my closeness with the trans and LGBTQ communities prior to the research troubles an insider/outsider binary, particularly as it was during the research that I explicitly articulated my own non-binary gender identity. Researcher involvement can necessitate becoming an insider with particular forms of ethnographic study, such that the study of community also allows autoethnography (Crossley, 2006; Throsby, 2016). While I would not position this research as inherently and essentially 'creating' my identity, it arguably produced an effective environmental circumstance for transformative reflection on identity (Ganga and Scott, 2006; Breen, 2007). By being reflexively conscientious of my own positionality in relation to the subject matter, I aim to sharpen my appreciation of factors that shaped the production of the analysis (Kanuha, 2000). Further, working from a position as an insider has multiple recognised advantages, as was demonstrated by my relative ease regarding recruitment and rapport (LaSala, 2003).

Conclusion

The methodological basis of this work aimed to privilege the ability of non-binary voices to tell new stories (Plummer, 1995). I have descriptively grounded and clarified how fieldwork was done, and laid the theoretical foundations that situated mixed-media diaries and semi-structured interviews in relation to each other, and to the project overall. I have fully elucidated the decisions made to successfully recruit participants, to develop and sustain rapport, and most importantly to ensure rigorous ethical safeguarding. The methodological decision to construct a multi-method project was made use of in my analytical practices, as the ability to begin the coding of diaries gave greater security in the ability of interviews to cover material deemed salient by participants.

Recognising additional demographic dimensions of participants was important in avoiding positioning consideration of gender identity in a social vacuum. Demographic similarities (such as age) and differences (such as race) to prior non-binary-specific research samples (Harrison et al., 2012) may be understood in relation to method limitations, the demographic make-up of the UK overall, and who may be more or less likely to be able to articulate a non-binary identity and be accessible to research.

While no work is without its limitations, I have argued how my choice of methods served to produce data in an effective way, while also being compatible with an emancipatory trans politics. Rejecting a positivist approach and drawing on symbolic interactionism within social constructionism (Jackson and Scott, 2010), this combination of framework, methods and analysis has allowed for a process of collaborative knowledge production, with resultant analysis illustrative of synergy between researcher and participants. The contents of diaries and interviews provides some of the first data to consider non-binary identities as a discrete yet amorphous set of realities, negotiating social and medical differences or needs. The following chapters will detail and analyse central themes identified within the data.

Notes

1   Jackson and Scott draw on Gagnon and Simon's (1974) work *Sexual Conduct* in considering these three categories as the key divisions of 'scripting', that is 'the application of sociocultural scripts that imbue [objects] with meaning' (Jackson and Scott, 2010: 814). Cultural interactions are had between the individual and social structures, such as a government. The interpersonal indicates those interactions that occur between an actor and other individuals, while the intrapsychic is when an individual introspects, viewing the self from a third person perspective.

2   Also called ME – myalgic encephalomyelitis.

3   While this was a beneficial decision due to the insights that were generated, this particular poem was not used in later analysis due to space constraints and overall fit with discussed themes.

4   For any reader interested in looking at any of these documents, they comprise the appendices to the 2016 thesis this book is based on. The thesis is freely available for download at: http://etheses.whiterose.ac.uk/15956/.

5   I am grateful to Teela Sanders and Karen Throsby who oversaw this process and made these recommendations with a feminist ethic of pedagogic care.

6   These posts are no longer publicly available – I felt compelled to remove them due to the rise in hostility towards trans and gender diverse people and their allies in public discourse, such that risks associated with sharing of one's personal narrative feels heightened. I retain these now-vulnerable early texts privately, and draw on them in my reflections here.

7   By this, I mean with their gender identity, cisness and so on. Many works use autobiography to enrich scholarship in other gendered contexts. For a classic example intersecting with class analysis, see Steedman (1987).

8   In Chapter 4 I discuss both Jen and Frankie as examples of identity shifts from 'non-binary to binary'. Prior to the interview Frankie had told me that they/them pronouns were correct. In the interview, Frankie talked about becoming "very grounded" in "a non-conforming female identity", and how while they still identified as non-binary "to a small extent", they also talked about non-binary identification in the past tense. This raises an ethical question about whether to infer use of she/her pronouns for Frankie throughout. I have elected not to, as I believe the assertion of power through taking the liberty of pronoun assumption as a researcher is best avoided. I have no way of ultimately knowing whether 'she/her' became the correct pronoun for Frankie, or when, or, if so, if this is still the case. I can only apologise to any participant where the 'pronoun snapshot' has aged beyond accuracy.

9   Both 'she' and 'they' pronouns are used throughout the book for Jess as she specified appreciating variation.

3

'Not trans enough': the relationship between non-binary gender identities, uncertainty and legitimacy

> Using queerness itself as a category of analysis seems to invite a new round of debate devoted to who is 'really queer'. A voice that originated from one set of margins begins to create its own marginalized voices. These twin problems of identities – boundaries and hierarchies – emerge whenever we try to base politics on identity. (Wilchins, 2002: 29)

Introduction

Among non-binary people, there is a vast heterogeneity of experiences and self-conceptualisations. Despite such differences, a striking commonality was observed among participants: insecurity in relation to gender. This could manifest as an internal uncertainty over whether one was 'trans enough', or fear of not being seen as trans enough by other people. This chapter will explore this phenomenon, while considering how hegemonic gendered expectations affect not only the ability to socially exert, but to internally formulate a non-binary gender identity. This exploration cuts across the original research questions, as feelings of insecurity were manifested in relation to experiences of queer community interaction, everyday experiences and accessing (or concern over accessing) medical support. Further, introspection was, perhaps predictably, strongly influenced by societal gender norms (both within and outside queer communities), which could be internalised, resisted, or both simultaneously.

I begin by highlighting how non-binary people who had not accessed gender-affirming medical services could view those who had as 'more legitimate' than themselves, even if they did not want such access. Critically, participants didn't view *others* who weren't medically transitioning as less legitimate. Rather, they held themselves to different standards of validity, highlighting how the anxiety of 'realness' often operated at the level of the self. Participants were self-aware and critical of such feelings as problematic. This may be suggestive of difficulties with, or low self-esteem in relation to, gender identity (Neff, 2003).

I then argue that hegemonic medicalised narratives of what it 'means to be transgender' have shaped queer community interactions. I show how community tensions can manifest with regards to non-binary people being made to feel 'not trans enough' by other members of trans communities. Binary-oriented trans people could sometimes exhibit hostility towards particular identities, or construct implicit hierarchies of legitimacy in order to self-validate. Such practices serve to evidence the problematic nature of processes where trans/non-binary identities are often only validated (by doctors, the law, family or friends, or in day-to-day social interactions) once difficult or painful processes have been navigated or performed. These include, but are not limited to, vocal and repeat performances of 'coming out', name changes and altering gendered presentation, as well as accessing hormones and surgeries. Of course, these are all often desirable and beneficial, yet can be problematised when expected (especially if expected in a particular way).

Participants also voiced anxieties over not being seen as trans enough when accessing (or wishing to access) gender-affirming medical services. This was navigated by some participants by presenting themselves to clinicians as 'simply' trans men or women, or by discussing their non-binary experiences of gender in binary terms in order to render themselves more compatible with clinical precedent. This affected the support individuals sought from queer community networks, and correspondingly shaped strategies of empowerment, resistance and navigation of medical services.

Impact of a binarised medical narrative on non-binary feelings of validity

As outlined in Chapter 1, hegemonic Western transgender narratives were constructed and constrained through processes of medical gatekeeping. Whether a participant wished to access gender-affirming medicine or not was significant in shaping how gender was considered.

Ben:	'Have you ever had feelings of not being trans enough?'
Jess:	'Yeah, all the time [laughs]. I think partially it's because I don't really feel a great need to access hormones or surgery. That I ... don't, I often feel like I'm some sort of fraud. Operating within this woman's space – or within a trans space because I don't really ... I'm not

really that bothered about changing my body. I kind of feel like my body is my body? And that it is what it is. I wouldn't be against changing it, but on balance it's probably more effort to change it than not to. Maybe that balance will shift over the years, especially if my hair decides to fall out, I might be more interested in taking hormones or whatever. But essentially because of my ambivalence towards these medical interventions, I do feel like I'm often not trans enough. And especially as somebody who's working in trans healthcare, as an activist and on the scene, I feel like people often expect me to be wanting to engage or be going on some sort of binary transition pathway or something like that. Sometimes I do think, what am I doing here, why am I claiming trans, why am I claiming womanhood, why am I claiming non-binary when I'm not particularly interested in changing my body? But being called he, being called my birth name, whatever, does make me feel uncomfortable. So, I do have some form of dysphoria, but it doesn't seem to be as soul destroying as a lot of people's physical dysphoria can be.' (Jess, 26, interview)

Jess felt that her ambivalence over her embodiment had produced self-doubt, due to the centrality and ubiquity of embodied dysphoria[1] narratives. It is also apparent that different aspects of embodiment hold differing levels of significance, as evidenced by her feeling that (male pattern) baldness would likely cause 'the balance to shift'. Hair and hairstyles function as significant sites through which gender can be socially enacted. How this particular gendered and embodied trait shifts over time was positioned as potentially altering Jess's broader decisions regarding embodiment. This diverges from both a historic model where pathologised distress was deemed necessary to be understood as trans, and from gatekeeping contemporary practices which emphasise trans people's 'individual clinical need but not their personal social preference' (NHS England cited in Pearce, 2018: 93). When articulating oneself sincerely runs against decades of the 'wrong-body model' of transness (Bettcher, 2014) it is intuitive for this to stimulate insecurity even when disidentifying with one's assignment at birth, due to the relative power of these discourses. It is a challenge to shake off the impact of clinical conceptions of trans being, even when one is active in deconstructing and rejecting such a paradigm.

Discursive relations between medical practice and communities are not a one-way street. Clinicians have slowly adapted and responded to the growth and change they have seen in the individuals accessing care. The criteria of the 10th revision of the International Statistical Classification of Diseases and Related Health Problems (ICD-10), characterise 'Transsexualism' (under the rubric of 'Gender identity disorders') as comprising 'The desire to live and be accepted as a member of the opposite sex, usually accompanied by the wish to make his or her body as congruent as possible with the preferred sex through surgery and hormone treatment' (WHO, 2016). The 11th revision[2] instead defines 'Gender incongruence of adolescence and adulthood' as:

> [C]haracterized by a marked and persistent incongruence between an individual's experienced gender and the assigned sex, which often leads to a desire to 'transition', in order to live and be accepted as a person of the experienced gender, through hormonal treatment, surgery or other health care services to make the individual's body align, as much as desired and to the extent possible, with the experienced gender. (WHO, 2016)

Charlie articulated a related concern in their diary – 'A brief thought – am I still trans if I don't want to transition?' – further emphasising that the approach to understanding what trans *is* remains connected to an assumed desire for medical transition, even among non-binary people. This is particularly conceivable for individuals in the early stages of exploring their gender identities, who are less likely to have experienced the rich community discourses of what trans and non-binary can be taken to mean. Alex discussed how meeting a particular partner was the first time they had knowingly met a trans person:

> This person is choosing not to socially transition for their own personal reasons, but I hadn't known you could do that. I kind of thought it was all or nothing? You know how you get that trope of like uneducated people saying 'oh have you had the operation yet?' And that was kind of my understanding of it until I got to know more people. (Alex, 20, diary)

Alex's experience illustrates how connecting with other trans/non-binary people can expand an individual's potentiality of gendered self-conception, through accessing discourses previously unknown to them. This also shows how Alex's present position (in relation to knowledge and community) means that they associate their past-self as 'uneducated', rather than merely inexperienced. Further, it emphasises the importance of interpersonal interactions to gain knowledge and awareness about non-binary/trans communities, which can have an impact on the intrapsychic interactions that allow for negotiation of the self.

Communities can share politicised knowledge that resists hegemonic positioning of homogeneous, historic narratives of coming out, and both social and medical transitions. For example, when individuals explore communities for the first time, they may be introduced to deconstructions of maleness and femaleness, in order to help reassure individuals of the validity of their identities. An example would be Jess recounting experiences of dysphoria that are not (especially) situated in the body, resisting an essentialised model of trans-being and allowing for different possibilities of gendered narratives. This however may then lack intelligibility within clinical settings. Hal made the point that trans communities are more common and conceptually recognisable than specifically non-binary communities.[3] Finding similar individuals with whom to bond or receive support over identity negotiation may therefore begin more generally, and become more specific over time as relationships are developed. Indeed, Alex demonstrated this through admitting their comparative ignorance when first interacting with other trans people.

While the 'classic' narrative of trans people being considered as men or women 'trapped in the wrong body' has been critically deconstructed (Bettcher, 2014), Rachel subverts the hegemonic interpretation that this produces uncomplicated, negative feelings. This is illustrated by Figure 2, taken from Rachel's diary.

Rachel's diary was digitally produced, and comprised entirely of short passages of text overlaid on images that were thematically connected to the context of the text as a multi-media form of expression. While Rachel does experience embodied dysphoria, in articulating that they find their body 'comfy and pretty and safe' they challenge a narrative that constructs trans bodies as exclusively problematic and negative for the trans individual. There is however still a degree of disjunction between self and body – 'it looks after me', rather than 'it *is* me'.

Rachel also highlights the importance of recognising trans people who have (at least partially) positive relationships with their bodies prior to, or without, hormonal and surgical changes. The image of lips wearing red lipstick, with the teeth biting the bottom lip is open

Figure 2: Image from Rachel's diary

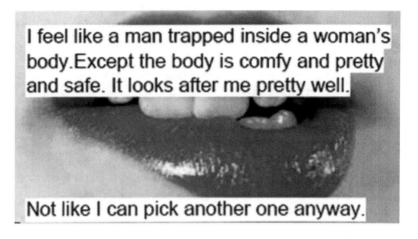

to a wide possibility of interpretations. While the lipstick may incite the viewer to instinctively gender the lips as female/feminine, the accompanying text allows for the reflexive reinterpretation of the image – recognising the fact that there is no available information to make a confident attribution of gender to the disembodied lips. There is concordance between text and image in that both challenge assumptions that might be made in relation to gendered discourse. The biting of the bottom lip has a cultural connotation of a sort of 'sexy coyness', though also has an association with anxiety or stress, or a sense of known misbehaviour. I interpret the image choice as connected to the text as a form of confessional, a semi-private admission that their sense of themselves deviates from the classic trope due to the positive and ambivalent notes. While a slightly subtle example, I argue non-binary people are acutely aware of the challenges that rendering themselves as real pose across clinical, community and practical contexts. To borrow a phrase from Gill and Elias (2014), there is a paradox of realness – a sense of self-knowledge contrasted with social unknowability. The weight of this may explain differing mechanisms of self-reassurance – Jess's social dysphoria, Alex's attention to what others are doing while asserting themselves as trans, Rachel's partial resonance with the classic trans concept.

Finn experienced uncertainty related to gender in different terms. While Charlie doubted their trans modality due to not feeling a need to access gender-affirming medical services, Finn doubted their *right* to access medical transition services on the basis of not possessing a binary gender identity:

> Too often I fall into the trap of thinking 'well I don't identify as a man so I shouldn't really be medically transitioning' but that's ridiculous. Just because I don't fit nicely into a binary trans narrative, doesn't mean that I shouldn't be able to get access to a body I will be much more comfortable in and that will align more with my inner image of what I actually look like, so that I'll be able to navigate the world and people will really see me. (Finn, 22, diary, emphasis original)

Finn's description of what they hope for from medical transition resonates with historically traditional binary-oriented trans narratives, which position the 'inner image' as stable and constant. Non-binary and binary-oriented trans motivations for transition may thus be similar – yet potentially still broader than medical hegemony is comfortable with recognising (Baril and Trevenen, 2014).

Ash was the only participant to explicitly state that, at this stage of their life, they never felt 'not trans enough', stating "I'm about as trans as most people get!" This was related to Ash's extensive history of accessing hormones and a wide range of gender-affirming surgeries. It is notable that this feeling was dynamic. In having altered their body, Ash fulfilled the requirements of a problematic yet totemic discourse of trans legitimisation. Surgery may then serve to provide even greater feelings of legitimacy than hormone access, due to being seen as more major (in terms of risk, cost, 'seriousness' and so on) – and having a history of being 'the ultimate goal', the transformative event (Plemons, 2019). Ash's diary included a self-portrait of their body, acting as a physical map of embodied change, and also a rough timeline of their gender-related medical interventions (Figure 3).

Ash had by far the most experience of surgical interventions among all participants. Extensive engagement with medical services synergised with long-term involvement with queer communities to result in strong feelings of legitimacy and validity for Ash in relation to being both transgender and non-binary.

It is important to note that while some participants expressed discomfort with aspects of their bodies and others did not, the general idea that accessing a medical transition allows one to be viewed as more authentically trans cut across these different non-binary experiences. Further, some participants, such as Finn, would challenge their own feelings as problematic and remind themselves of political arguments that trans status need not rest on embodied dysphoria. This bears a striking overlap with findings by Catalano (2015) who found that a

Figure 3: Image from Ash's diary

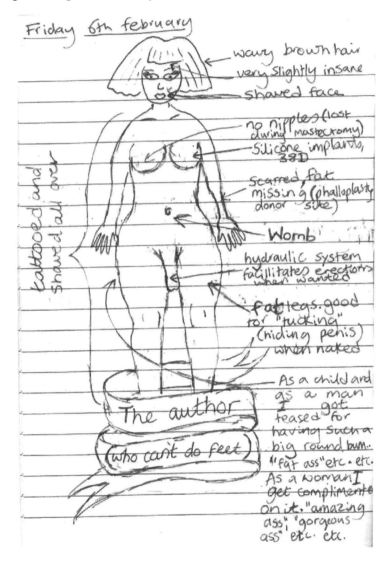

sample of trans male undergraduate students could rely on medical discourse, even while critiquing it. In this passage, Jamie connected their insecurity to their frustration with the relationship between narrative performed and respect/understanding received:

> I knew I wasn't female but thought I couldn't be "really trans" because I hadn't experienced dysphoria etc. consistently for long enough ... of course I'm both

non-binary and trans, if you have to see them as separate things which I don't believe you should (I tend to think you're either cis or not cis). It drives me mad how well that story of repression and "coming to terms with" my trans identity and going through a 'NB stage' works: it reaffirms everything that's wrong with the way people think about gender. It drives me mad too, that when people hear it, they're super relieved to be able to use male pronouns for me and never have to deal with these pesky gender-neutral ones again. And it drives me maddest of all that experience keeps proving that that story is the only way to get people to take my seriously, to actually try hard with pronouns, to pay more than lip service to the pain being misgendered causes me. (Jamie, 24, diary)

This illustrates again how an uncertain relationship with dysphoria of the body troubled their ability to embrace a trans identity. The language around dysphoria not being 'consistent' or for 'long enough' resembles a medicalised consideration of the assessment of symptoms in relation to illness. Individuals are thus more likely to feel insecure of the 'validity' of their gender identities when less certain that they are fulfilling medically validated discourses of transgender.

In addition, Jamie's relationship with pronouns (preferring singular they, but also accepting 'he', at the time) meant that in circumstances where explanations of 'they' as their pronoun might be too difficult – that is, emotionally exhausting or posing a risk of disenfranchisement, ridicule or violence – they possessed an intelligible and personally acceptable option. Jess also navigated gendered interactions similarly, using both 'they' and 'she', though without particular preference. She pointed out:

> 'I give "she" or "they" as pronouns. And I say use them equally, I pretty much exclusively within the trans community get called she. And this is because I think even if trans people were … we want to be in the binary or want to put people in the binary.' (Jess, 26, interview)

Jamie and Jess's narratives show how constructing an understanding of dysphoria that is broader than a medicalised perspective resting on the body, allows for a sense of validation and inclusion. By constructing their negative feelings of being misgendered as a distinct form of dysphoria (rather than catalysing embodied dysphoria), this utilises clinical language to challenge and resist any internal sense of inadequacy or fraudulence.

Jess's example emphasises that even in trans communities, binarised language may be leaned into when the choice is given. This emphasises the potential difficulty in navigating being non-binary and intelligible, even in queer spaces. The sense of feeling 'trans enough' was not rooted exclusively in internal policing or insecurity, with some participants reflecting on how community interactions could foster or stimulate a sense of not belonging.

Hierarchy of transness within trans communities

Jen expressed feeling that while labels had helped her to articulate her identity, they could also make her feel like an outsider. Her relationship with trans further illustrates the connection between feeling trans enough and medical transition, while introducing how those feelings can impact interactions within trans communities:

> I often feel like an outsider among trans people because I can't transition. So if I'm in Girl Mode and I choose to present as female, and I'm with a bunch of transwomen, I feel like the odd one out. Transwomen are usually transitioning or have transitioned. Of course they are. They aren't drag queens (no offense to drag queens). If I'm not transitioning, am I really a transwoman? I guess the answer is no. I'm a guy in woman's clothes, which isn't the same thing. I don't think that's entirely true (I don't feel like a guy at the time) but that's how I feel in terms of being an outsider. (Jen, 29, diary)

At the time of the research Jen identified as bigender, experiencing her gender as shifting between what she termed 'boy mode' and 'girl mode'. Jen expressed that she cannot medically transition, because she felt that while she would want physiological traits associated with being female when in 'girl mode', she would want her body to remain as it is when in 'boy mode', such that no physiological configuration would be satisfying at all times.[4] An androgynous or mix of physiological traits would also not be what Jen wanted, as she understood her gender in distinctly bimodal terms. Experiencing gender differently from (medically constructed and validated) narratives of transgender caused Jen to doubt her 'transness'. This echoes Charlie's insecurity over being trans if not transitioning. Jen was among several participants who articulated a sense of a 'trans hierarchy' within queer community spaces, between those accessing or wishing to access medical transition services and those not:

> I still get some problems from some trans people, but in this comment I'm meaning more people who are understanding loosely what trans is and are okay with Caitlyn Jenner,[5] they're like 'what are you then, because you're obviously not a trans woman'. You're just faking it, or not sure? (Jen, 29, diary)

Jen's articulation of a bigender identity meant that she felt that, by the standards of those interacting with her, she was 'obviously not a trans woman'. Feeling confronted with questions such as 'you're faking it, or not sure?' within trans communities illustrates that there is not always an equivalent sense of awareness, acceptance or sensitivity towards non-binary people. Those trans individuals who most closely fulfil historic clinical expectations of what being transgender 'is' are those also positioned as 'most sure' or 'most real' within some trans communities. Binary-oriented trans people[6] are thus positioned as less likely to be viewed as 'faking it or not sure' than non-binary people, in Jen's view. However, discourses of binary-oriented trans women as 'gender deceivers', particularly as a form of transmisogyny, have been recognised and explored (Serano, 2007). Further, community members' feelings on transgender hierarchies of authenticity have been previously recognised (Hines, 2007a), with participants reporting a need for trans communities to move beyond such practices.

Even when not being seen as trans enough was not a factor, anxiety over other community members' thoughts could affect how participants felt, affecting their experiences of queer communities:

Ben: 'Have you ever had feelings of not being trans enough?'

Frankie: 'Oh lord yes. Oh lord yes. I think I have to be honest – hormones were a really validating experience in that sense. Prior to hormones, I had those feelings constantly. That was a real demon that I was battling for a long time. There is a hierarchy of transness amongst trans communities, there just is. And it's really damaging and really hurtful and really horrible.'

B: 'In that people are seen more real when they access medical services?'

F: 'Abso-fucking-lutely. And whether there's been an internalisation of that I think it's pretty apparent there has.' (Frankie, 25, interview)

Frankie's experience of medicine as validating re-emphasises how their experience prior to accessing medicine felt less stable, that they felt more vulnerable to being seen as invalid or illegitimate by other trans people. Rachel's diary also emphasises how insecurity due to not accessing a medical transition need not only be rooted in ambivalence towards embodied changes, but may well illustrate important considerations such as how disabilities may intersect with accessibility or the desirability of medical transition. This discussion is expanded in Chapter 5. David illustrated a different connection between medicine and insecurity over being accepted as trans:

Ben: 'Have you ever had feelings of not being trans enough?'
David: 'Oh god, all of the time.'
B: 'What causes that?'
D: 'I think largely, the lack of any medical transition, ultimately the only thing people have to go on with me describing myself as trans is my word. I have no evidence for it whatsoever. Not even ... I don't even have any official documents in the name that I go by, because I've changed my name a couple of times now and it's a hassle and I can't be arsed. And because I think that I might be in 'name transition' at the moment? So I might yet change it again. And I don't want to have to go through the entire process again. So yeah, but it is mostly the medical stuff that makes me feel like ... I think if I was on hormones no one would ever question it.' (David, 31, interview)

It is worth recognising how David's use of language – not having 'evidence' of their transness – mirrors that of evidence-based medicine, sometimes concerning itself with 'proof' to legitimise an individual's identity (for example, evidence of so-called 'real life experience' of gender as a prerequisite for surgery). The medical establishment has both direct and indirect roles in the production of transgender narratives, and how these may affect individual conceptualisation and expression of self. Further, while even clinical sites of knowledge production are increasingly explicit that being trans is neither an illness nor a disorder (Richards et al., 2015), this can fail to adequately recognise how practices of treatment access are rooted in and (re) produce discourses about trans in the same way *as if* dis-identification with assignment at birth were a pathology.

Finn stated how they felt the view of not feeling trans enough due to not accessing medical services could be reinforced through the beliefs of some binary-oriented trans people:

> I think there's a lot of problems in trans communities of like, oh well if you're not dysphoric then you can't be trans, like being non-binary isn't a thing, non-binary people don't belong in trans communities. (Finn, 22, diary)

This adds traction to the ways in which Jess and Jamie constructed their feelings of discomfort over being misgendered and deadnamed[7] through the language of dysphoria specifically. By articulating distress in relation to language as dysphoria, this justifies inclusion under the trans umbrella to those who may attempt to police boundaries of transness in terms of distress and discomfort. Inclusion through a rubric of suffering might be framed as, to borrow Natalie Wynn's (2018: timestamp: 30:10) phrase, 'masochistic epistemology' – "whatever hurts is true". While Wynn was using this to refer to a tendency to dismiss compliments and internalise insults, in this context it might be reformulated as 'being trans/non-binary must hurt to be *real*' – masochistic ontology.

Mark's view of trans communities was that some individuals could validate themselves through reliance on comparison to other community members, such that some individuals would justify their identity though an exclusionary politics of realness. When asked if there could be conflict in community settings, Mark answered:

Mark: 'Oh absolutely. I mean even in our little group, we have like eight to ten people along, I don't think I'm breaking any confidences here when I say for some, they identify in a very binary way, and that's how they're going through their transition, that's how they are knitting everything together for themselves. And we have probably two or three people ... in addition to myself who would probably identify as non-binary, and it can be sometimes that ... it's not so much conflict, as I say, we're drinking cups of tea and eating Victoria sandwich, so there's not going to be any pitched battles, but there is a bit of one-upmanship almost. [...] everybody's I suppose ... trying to kind of ... grab the label for themselves; that makes it seem very conscious, and I don't think it is. But we all want to be right, don't we [...] In the kind of "transgender world"... there's such a kind of chorus of people who are singing more or less the same song, off a similar sort of hymn sheet, but maybe using a different key! None of which is wrong. And that, well, very little of which is probably wrong, but that's where the trouble comes, it's very difficult to say to somebody else, "I'm sorry, you're wrong about your transition," you can't say you're non-binary for reason X Y Z.'

Ben: 'Well there's never any reason to do that.'

M: 'I would hope not, but I think sometimes in the mission to find ourselves we kind of do it by stomping on other people, either deliberately or not.' (Mark, 43, interview)

V discussed how he views it as important that those with 'normative' trans identities and experiences do not 'set a standard' for gender-diverse communities:

'I've certainly heard it, and I think [hierarchies in trans communities are] a bit insidious in some of the groups without being overt; you get a feeling certain people switch off when you start being a bit more nuanced about it. Because all they're bothered about is being read as blah. As a stereotype, and that's it. And then they want to get on with their lives. And they're not really interested in the nuance of identity; they just want to be comfortable and not hassled, which is fair enough. But again, that sort of thing is not helpful to the community at large. If that's how you want to be, that's fine. But don't make that the structure of transness, or the social acceptance of transness. Interestingly, I recently came across someone who said they'd got hassle as quite a binary trans person for being binary, from people who were non-binary! And I have honestly never heard that before [...] normally it's the other way around [...] So that was quite interesting because a little part of me felt that perhaps they'd said that because they felt a little bit, I don't know, insecure about people being non-binary. And that's sort of the impression I got from them as a person, talking to them. That their identity was

affirmed in a very binary way and so being non-binary they kind
of didn't connect with, and felt a little bit threatened by, perhaps,
or just not comfortable with it. Which you know, is alright but
it's a bit ... to kind of promote that socially is uncomfortable, I
think.' (V, 28, interview)

V argues that it is important for trans people not to articulate
their validity and self-affirmation through the denigration of other
people's gender identities and expressions. Non-binary people will
be inherently disadvantaged in any situation where individuals appeal
to historically legitimised trans narratives as more certain, real or
stable, as it is only relatively recently that non-binary identities have
been recognised within policy and medical practice. The logic of
masochistic ontology when deployed to delegitimise others (for their
seeming lack of pain, or lack of appropriately severe and unambiguous
pain) can be connected to gatekeeping in clinical contexts. Access to
gender-affirming medical interventions in the UK via the NHS hinges
on an assessment, yielding a diagnosis. Fear of being found insufficient,
or a need to remind oneself that one has been 'accepted' may require
buying into the logic of gatekeeping practice: that *compos mentis* adults
desirous of gender-affirming medical interventions exist but for whom
this would be supposedly 'inappropriate'– a premise necessary to
accept for assessment to be justified. Accepting such a rationale may
allow an individual to better tolerate their own assessment, while
discursively encouraging community practices where pain signifies
one's right to belong.

Trans rights have a cultural and legal history of being hard-won.
Thus, inclusion of individuals under the trans umbrella who have
identities and/or gender expressions that challenge the gender binary
and cisnormative hegemony may sensitise or even anger those binary-
oriented trans people who possess more conservative beliefs regarding
the ontology or operation of gender. This suggestion is borne out
through Jamie's description of interactions with some members of
a trans support/social group they attend. Jamie contextualises by
describing a particular older trans woman as regularly interrupting
others and dominating discussions. She was characterised as
conservative, causing tensions with some younger members who
problematise such a worldview. Jamie explains how:

'[She] not last night, but the time before, went on a rant about
the word "queer" – because it was used as an insult when she
was young. And said "and there's this booklet over there which

says you can identify as 'genderqueer', and I want to rip it up!"
and my friend who identifies as genderqueer got really upset and
said "You can't do that, you're erasing people's identity," and at
that point I would have wanted someone in charge to step in
and say "Just to remind people, everyone has the right to identify
how they like," but they didn't. People who were nominally in
charge were just sitting in the corner awkwardly and this really
quite heated discussion going on. And [she was] interrupting
everyone, expressing this unpleasantly privileged way of socially
interacting.' (Jamie, 24, interview)

Tensions regarding the reclamation of language and how that has
become incorporated into identity politics can illustrate not only a
lack of understanding but catalyse hostility that can be difficult to
manage. This example illustrates the possibility of heterogeneous
community spaces as disputatious. There is potential for trans
people whose validation has been achieved within normative
terms to exercise community surveillance and to sanction non-
normative behaviour. This may be compared with homonormative
policing, particularly within communities of gay and bisexual men
(Taywaditep, 2002).

Jess considers the difficulty in disconnecting a trans identity
from a medical transition to be the product of medical
institutionalisation, exerting a hegemonic binary of medical-transition-
versus-cisgender:

'I think transness has kind of been stolen from us really. There's
a whole wide range of gender experience that you could classify
as being trans. And I think that what has happened is those
experiences have been pathologised by the medical establishment
and been forced into a psychopathologised binary medical
pathway. Which forces you to be essentially a binary trans
person, or forces what is essentially a spectrum to become a
yes or no question. And so, I wouldn't want to put that on the
queer community, I don't think that's a queer community ... I
think we're living under the shadow of that rather than creating
it. But I think there's a few things that we do which perpetuates
the 'common sense' we've received from above. So we often
expect people to want to engage in medical interventions. We
often expect a certain type of presentation. We expect people
to operate in those kind of ways. So yeah. I think that there's
stuff that the queer community could be working on within

themselves as well as engaging with non-queer community.'
(Jess, 26, interview)

Jess's explanation shifts the focus of critique away other members of trans communities who may perpetuate dominant narratives by operating relatively easily within medical diagnostic paradigms. Instead, Jess emphasises how gender-diverse communities 'live under a shadow' of medicalisation which is responsible for intra-community policing, as well as internalisation of not feeling trans enough relative to service access. This shifts the modality of oppression away from individuals within a marginalised population, and towards the structural constraints of the medical establishment, and the discourses which its processes reinforce.

Feeling not trans enough in relation to medical service access

There was a sense among participants that non-binary gender identities could lack cultural intelligibility even within trans communities. This was dwarfed by concerns over whether GIC medical practitioners would be affirming, or aware of non-binary identities – despite supposed specialisation/expertise. Multiple participants articulated that they felt binarised medical gatekeeping is a common occurrence, and would prevent their non-binary trans status from being legitimised if they were entirely candid.

> Have I therefore made up my gender story? Yes, a bit, to concrete the impression I've given to my doctors. But not in the essentials. (Mark, 43, diary)

> I've been having a lot of very difficult feelings surrounding my gender, mainly due to knowing how hard it is for non-binary people to get treated at Gender Identity Clinics, and wondering if I should lie and say I'm a trans guy (which I probably will end up doing). (Finn, 22, diary)

Ash: 'I think it is [different for non-binary people to access GICs]. Because when you go into an exchange with a medical professional who's assessing you for some sort of treatment, you ... probably have if not a certainty about what you want to do, at least the idea that you don't want to actively cut off your options by admitting that you're not a trans binary person. Because once they decide that they've assessed you and you're not transsexual you definitely won't get any hormones et cetera so there's a defensiveness and a realisation that if you go in and let them know how uncertain you are or how non-binary you are that you'll just cut off all your options for the future. I think a lot of us, if we don't lie, we really deliberately present all the stuff that makes a good case for treatment because that's what we want to do, and we can always change our mind and not have the treatment. But once they've said no to the treatment, we can't change our minds about that, not too easily. So that's what makes it difficult to be honest.'

B: 'So, do you think people try to keep their options open by presenting more binary than they maybe are?'

A: 'Yes, I think so. More binary, more certain. More ... yeah. Absolutely. More like ... the narrative of 'typical transsexual' experiences known to have worked.' (Ash, 33, interview)

There is a sense among non-binary people that medical practices create disparity for non-binary individuals regarding validation and access to interventions. Ash explained how when they accessed hormones and surgeries initially, they identified as a binary-oriented trans man, and then had great difficulty in accessing further services in relation to their articulation of a non-binary identity. They explained how:

'When I went on the waiting list for breast surgery, I imagined that I wasn't actually going to have it. I did it because it was expected of me, and if I did everything that was expected of me, I'd get a prescription for testosterone. And I imagined I'd probably just go 'Oh I changed my mind' and not having it done.' (Ash, 33, interview)

However, Ash found the experience of 'becoming more butch' very interesting, and explained how their curiosity over being read socially as male resulted in continued medical access, which they felt positively about. These factors together also strongly influenced how they constructed their body outside a clinical setting, articulating how through extensive exercise they cultured a muscular, masculine physique. Despite enjoying this period of their life, after ten years

Ash decided they wanted to articulate a more feminine appearance. Negotiating this with medical professionals was extremely difficult, with Ash explaining that as they didn't follow a 'typical' trans narrative. They were turned away by at least ten surgeons before finding a private doctor in Poland willing to give Ash breast implants, despite having previously accessed a double mastectomy. Ash expressed an unambiguous happiness about their (new) breasts. They were also happy during the period of their life where they possessed a muscular, masculine, post-mastectomy chest. This serves to disrupt a trans narrative where a physiological configuration associated with one side of the gender binary is anathema, while the other is idealised. Two points (that are often implicitly positioned as axiomatic) are challenged by this – first that gender, once 'truly' reflected on and understood, does not and cannot change. Second, that the presentation and articulation of gender that a person feels is right for them reflects the *whole* gendered self, rather than a part. This experience of embodiment illustrates potential 'fuzziness' around gender (Tauchert, 2002). In other words, Ash's shift in embodied desire does not evidence remorse for their time spent presenting as masculine, nor does it imply that the allowances for medical intervention were misplaced. This has significant ramifications for the conceptualisation of 'detransition'.

The desire and action of Ash to modify their body in relation to how they felt regarding gender at different stages in their life defies the expectations of gender identity clinics – that gender-affirming procedures should be permanent. This expectation is due to the 'common sense' (and ultimately cissexist) notion that if gendered desire is impermanent, it is 'less real', which shapes the standards that are considered ethical within medical practice. Thus, there is a lack of clinically intelligible narratives where individuals have continued transitioning, or retransitioned, without it being characterised as 'regret'. Ash's experience also emphasised how happiness with one's body is not only affected by the body itself and a sense of what one wants/needs, but intersecting material factors also. Ash was a sex worker, and thus embodiment for them was also intimately connected to economic capital. It is also clear from Ash's narrative that they did not approach medical services attempting to articulate a binary-oriented trans narrative while identifying as non-binary, but rather came to their non-binary identification over time, post-medical access.

The presence of an assessment process that determines whether medical interventions can be accessed, and when (particularly through NHS GICs, though also through private medical practice), means that non-binary people may view certain narratives as more likely to 'succeed' than others:

Jamie: 'I think medically speaking, I don't think GICs would accept you just saying "this makes me happy, but I'm not super unhappy now".'

Ben: 'You have to be pathologically unhappy?'

J: 'Which is why again, you end up hyping up these experiences which maybe you would prefer to diminish. Because you're aware, or you think you're aware given there's no transparency, of what they want to hear. And you've got to strike a balance between telling that and telling the truth.' (Jamie, 24, interview)

Jess also explained their view that access to medical resources can become "a competition" as to who can fulfil clinical expectations "in the quickest and most attractive way". Jamie and Jess both share the view that current medical policy inherently produces a hierarchy between binary-oriented and non-binary trans people, because of the belief that non-binary identities are less likely to be accepted as *needing* treatment. One can argue that within the context of the NHS, while doctors are limited by available budgets, they nevertheless have a utilitarian responsibility for individuals who are experiencing pathological distress to be prioritised (Pencheon, 1998). This cannot be satisfactorily dissected without considering the ramifications of contemporary healthcare politics – such as competitive tendering, and in recent years, managing budgets under austerity – but this is beyond the scope of this work. However, as the multiple participants who experienced dysphoria and would be helped by gender-affirming medical services illustrate, patient need cannot be assessed through consideration of whether identity is constructed in binary-oriented or non-binary terms. Further, the existence of binary-oriented trans people who do not wish for hormones or surgeries has long been recognised, through the now defunct separation of 'transsexual' and 'transgender'. Historically, those not seeking medical transition could be clinically positioned as 'simply crossdressers', with this fundamental demarcation used to maintain 'transsexualism' as the only category necessitating medical transition, which required a particular performance of gender in order to be diagnosed as such.

It is important to recognise that doctors, like all members of society, are subject to influence by structural, societal gendered norms (Turner, 1995). Some participants feared being judged as 'not trans enough' by doctors because of being less culturally intelligible to them. There was a lack of confidence that one could reliably expect even basic sensitivity, even in specialist contexts, and concern that non-binary treatment[8] has considerably less precedent with which to be clinically justified. This is discussed in further detail in Chapters 5 and 6.

Frankie articulated positive feelings about their experiences at the GIC. Despite this, they added that their overall sense of *other* trans people's experiences was not good, and that there exists "a lot of misunderstanding, [and] a lot of barriers put up to [accessing] medical assistance". Other participants, who articulated positive experiences personally, also believed there was a negative status quo overall:

> You hear really awful stories, like, oh god, but that hasn't happened to me, I've been fortunate. (Mark, 43, diary)

> My non-binary friend, they've just been under the gender clinic, and they've had a really tough experience. And I think that's fairly typical from what I know. I have been incredibly lucky. (Ricky, 43, diary)

Frankie and Ricky's positive experiences are particularly important because they both identified themselves explicitly as non-binary to their GICs throughout their transition processes. Negative participant conceptions of GIC practice for non-binary people cannot be taken as universally representative, and as Frankie also notes, "you don't normally hear people being particularly vocal about the good experiences they've had, the ones you do hear about tend to be the negative ones". This follows, in that interactions perceived as problematic by gender-diverse communities inevitably garner more attention than positively experienced cases, in order to seek improvement. In addition, for those community members seeking information from other trans people prior to GIC access, interest in negative cases can be a motivated by a desire to avoid an undesirable outcome, preparing for a 'worst case scenario', learning about clinicians, and considering 'what not to do'. The above quotations suggest a pattern whereby non-binary people with positive clinical experiences view themselves as exceptions to the rule – "fortunate" and "lucky" – as they all had anecdotal evidence of problematic transgender treatment (at all levels of care) from others.

It is possible that Frankie's positive experience was connected to the manner in which they articulated their non-binary identity. They described themself to clinicians using simple, binarised language (such as 'more female than male'). Frankie even postulates that their experiences may have influenced how their identity changed over time from non-binary to more binary-oriented: "to be honest maybe that's part of the reason for my kind of identity shift. Maybe I wouldn't rule it out that I've internalised some … GIC". The potentiality of non-binary transition pathways being disciplined in a binary direction echoes Ash's experiences. This is not so crude as a literal insistence on binary identification, but that should a service user *happen* to experience such a process, this may be met with thinly veiled approval. Frankie reported that during one of their GIC appointments, one of their doctors said:

> That I was moving (I think the words he used were 'slowly drifting') towards a place that was much *easier to 'treat'* from the GIC's greater NHS perspectives because it had a treatment history. Much as I can understand this, it's a bit of a blow to hear it put like that. (Frankie, 25, diary, emphasis added)

By implying, therefore, that non-binary service users are 'more difficult' due to lack of historical precedent, it can be appreciated why non-binary people may feel the need to police how they communicate with GICs in order to make the process as quick and easy as possible for themselves. This is a product of a more general logic in medicine (of sign/symptom identification, diagnosis and treatment) being crudely applied in the context of gender, such that articulations of gender with less socially visible (and therefore medical) history are discursively positioned as having less medical need. This explains the commonality of some participants wishing to avoid or minimise mention of their non-binary identification within the GIC. Exhibiting a common and precedent-bearing profile could be done however, even if identifying oneself openly as non-binary. Ricky said that it was:

> 'Surprisingly easy [to be out as non-binary in medical contexts], but I think that I probably had enough of a typical trans man's narrative to make it a fairly straightforward process, even though … they were very respectful of my pronouns, and on my letter finally granting me testosterone has me recorded as a non-binary trans person, with 'they' pronouns. But having said that, I've gone on a fairly standard route. I'm going on testosterone, I have no desire at the moment for surgery, but that might change as my body changes. [...] So yeah, I don't know

whether my experience as a non-binary person in the gender clinic is typical of other non-binary people who might have slightly less standardised needs. I was talking, and toying with taking a lower dose of testosterone, which they're quite resistant to at [clinic]. But in the end, I decided to go for a full dose, just because the changes ... apparently if you take a lower dose of testosterone you get the same changes, just more slowly. And to be honest at my age, the changes will happen pretty slowly anyway.' (Ricky, 43, interview)

The language that Ricky used further emphasises the point that positive clinical experiences are positioned as something to be thankful for, rather than something that can be relied on. Ricky positioned the ease of being out as non-binary as 'surprising', though ameliorated this by suggesting this was through their clinical requests fitting within binary precedent – the "standard route".

Participants exerted control over their relationships with GICs through methods other than obscuring their non-binary identities, or through policing the manner in which they spoke about their identity. Despite both coming to this project independently and both electing to be anonymous, V and Jamie were open in their interviews about knowing each other and being friends. Jamie expressed how they had received support and advice from V, who had positive experiences of accessing a particular GIC. Jamie chose this clinic on the basis of V's recommendation, but still remained guarded:

I haven't self-defined as non-binary to the NHS. When I say I picked [clinic] because V says they're non-binary friendly, I mean I won't worry about going in in flowery shirts and earrings in both ears; that's all. That's the limit of my honesty – I'm just going to tell them I'm not female; that's not a lie. (Jamie, 24, diary)

The concern expressed by individuals accessing GICs goes beyond the desire to be respected and recognised by practitioners in the setting of consultation meetings – extending to contexts outside appointments, such as clinical forms. Jamie discusses and deconstructs this within their diary:

So this [clinic] form. 19 pages long. Includes a section where you label almost every body part with a rating of how you feel about it, including 'beard' (is that 'not satisfied', 'I want one', or N/A?) and <u>ears</u> (literally this has made me feel dysphoric about my ears, ffs).[9] A section on anxiety/depression, where you mark how often in the past week you've had a variety of anxious thoughts, which of course triggers all of said anxious thoughts. A section that seems designed to see if you have an eating disorder, with three slightly differently worded questions asking whether you think your buttocks are too big (if I say yes, will they think I just have an eating disorder and am not really trans?) And a section that maybe designed to test if you're autistic, I dunno – you have to rate the extent to which you agree with statements like "I would rather go to a library than a party" (is it a nice library? Who will be at the party? Did I get enough sleep the night before?) and most bizarrely "I find it easy to remember long strings of numbers, such as car number plates". That one caused a lot of anxiety at [group] because it sounds gender related inadvertently or not: 'masculine' brains are stereotypically supposed to remember numbers better. That's the problem with asking seemingly irrelevant questions in a context where there's so little trust between practitioners and patients: we start wondering why the questions are being asked, how they're relevant to the issue at hand, and what the "right answer" that will result in us getting access to treatment is. As if the process wasn't hoop-jump-y enough, and as if I didn't already feel obliged to lie about my NB identity, now I have to agonise over what ratio of library-to-party preference makes me trans enough. (Jamie, 24, diary, emphasis original)

There is a lack of transparency over how such forms are produced, why particular questions are included, and what particular purpose such questions serve; which as Jamie articulates, can cause experiences of anxiety over what criteria the GIC are attempting to scrutinise.[10] In the recent past, trans activists have given examples of service users being expected to completely comply with directions over gendered appearance and to obtain 'proof' of gender expression within the workplace (*PinkNews*, 2009) illustrating how GIC practices can discipline service users' genders, and how they choose to communicate.

The responses from Jamie's specific trans community in relation to this clinical form, which Jamie illustrates, raises the question of whether (and if so, to what extent) such questions on the clinical form are justified through evidence-based research. The inclusion of questions pertaining to 'systemising' ability – such as memorisation of car number places – may relate to theorisation within experimental psychology, postulating that brains are gendered male and female in and of themselves, which are then demarcated as 'systemising' and 'empathising' (Baron-Cohen, 2004).[11] This work has since been heavily criticised for containing fundamental methodological flaws and enforcing stereotypical notions of gender (Fine, 2010). Lack of transparency over the production of such forms also means it is unlikely that (or at least, unknown if) trans service users were consulted on their potential impact. There are also ethical implications should such data be used for research purposes, even with the informed consent of service users. Individuals may have feared being treated unfavourably, or feared denial of transition access should such forms not be fully completed – to not fulfil the role of a 'good patient' as optimally as possible. In any setting where access to gender-affirming medical interventions *can* be denied to an informed and mentally competent person, research enterprises will be fatally undermined.

This section has explored some perceptions and experiences of accessing gender-affirming medical services. Opinions on GIC sensitivity and their ability to treat non-binary people effectively were low, among those who had and had not accessed them. However, personal experiences *were* broadly positive – illustrating how it is possible that negative experiences may dominate community discourses, resulting in greater levels of anxiety and distrust. Alternatively, while interactions with clinicians may be broadly found to be satisfactory, the discourses regarding the clinic (that is, expectations of practitioner resistance or having to prove oneself as 'trans enough'), the lack of transparency, and anxiety over the *potential* of a distressing interaction limit how positively the clinic may be regarded. Further, the happiness and relief later experienced by individuals who are successful in accessing hormones and/or surgeries may potentially ameliorate more negative views they held at the time. Frankie's data is thus particularly interesting as they experienced a GIC appointment during their diary-keeping period.

It must also be noted that individuals with positive interactions in the clinical setting may still problematise the reasoning or efficacy of GIC policies or practices. While clinicians may be respectful and helpful, this can be recognised as occurring simultaneously with a lack of transparency, extensive waiting times (Vincent, 2018a), lack of universal clinic guidelines, and lack of non-binary protocols (Richards et al., 2016). Fear of being judged 'not trans enough' to access services is a serious concern for many, and relates to how communities have internalised a discourse which associates medical access with legitimacy. Thus, fear of rejection, delay or complication by medical providers may also be connected to fear of then being unable to be recognised as 'authentic' in community interactions. Medical transition services can emphasise that aspects of hormonal therapy and surgeries are permanent changes, and associate this with arriving at a static and fixed gender identity, which Ash's experience defies.

Conclusion

Throughout this chapter I have illustrated how common feelings of 'not being trans enough' can be among people with non-binary gender identities. This has significant discursive interplay with the consideration of, and interaction with, queer communities and medical services oriented to gender transition. Not feeling trans enough is commonly connected to either not desiring, or having not yet accessed medical services. This shows how the centrality of medical diagnoses and discourses to the history of trans communities shapes contemporary experiences of identity formation. This is despite resistance to medicalisation among trans/non-binary communities, and shifts in language among medical practitioners and diagnostic manuals over time, as recognised in Chapter 1. I have used the concept of 'embodied dysphoria' to differentiate between those who experience distress with their *bodies* and those who do not, and have drawn attention to how the language of dysphoria is used by non-binary individuals to justify themselves as trans, even while resisting the imposition of medical power.

In a report from the Scottish Trans Equality Network (Valentine, 2016c), non-binary participants who did not or were unsure about considering themselves trans expressed a range of reasons why. These included 'not feeling trans enough', but also 'not having changed gender presentation', 'not undergoing transition' (which may be broadly conceived as changing appearance, or more specifically referencing medical interventions), or because they felt the term 'only applied to binary-oriented trans men and women'. I argue that these four lines of reasoning can be subsumed under the broader sense of not feeling trans enough, as they are all examples of the *ways* in which people didn't feel trans enough. I assert that a belief in the right to the self-determination of gender is near-ubiquitous among the non-binary population, such that these reasonings only hold for the individual making them, and are not representative of a respondent having a prescriptive sense of what non-binary is, isn't, or should be. That is, a non-binary person who doesn't feel trans enough because they aren't accessing hormones is very unlikely to assert that *all* non-binary people who aren't accessing hormones are de facto not trans. There are some non-binary people whose reasons for not 'taking-up' trans are personal and/or political in ways that are not related to any sense that they 'cannot' because of something lacking. For example, some respondents to the Scottish survey said they felt trans as an identity category was too closely associated with the gender binary.

Tensions can sometimes manifest between members of trans communities, sometimes due to non-essential but clustered differences between binary-oriented and non-binary trans people. Reasons for this have included generational differences in language use, and how an understanding of one's own and other's genders are subject to many sociocultural factors, constructing what individuals perceive as valid or real. In some contexts, insecurity about one's gender may also lead to attempts at self-validation through the denigration of others, which is problematic and entwined – if not with medical access, then with suffering – which I frame as masochistic ontology. This can be at the particular expense of non-binary individuals; if a binary-oriented trans person adopts a medical paradigm to affirm themselves, non-binary identities are then correspondingly accorded less precedence, and greater association with uncertainty, indecision, impermanence, flux and difficulty to understand and/or 'treat'.

Notes

[1] I use the term 'embodied dysphoria' to refer to negative feelings that transgender people may experience specifically relating to their body itself – such as the presence or absence of primary or secondary sexual characteristics. I use this term to differentiate from social dysphoria – caused by interactions with other people, whereby the body is subjected to gendered interpretations which may be distressing (misgendering and so on).

[2] The version for implementation was first published June 2018, presented at the World Health Assembly in May 2019, and comes into effect January 2022.

[3] Though these certainly exist – an example being Non-Binary Leeds, which has links with Trans Leeds, but is separately organised. The groups have different but overlapping membership/attendance.

[4] After the project, Jen wrote to me, coming out as a trans woman. This dimension is considered in Chapter 4, having received explicit permission to include the correspondence in the project data.

[5] Caitlyn Jenner won the 1976 Olympic men's decathlon title, and established a television career most associated with 'Keeping up with the Kardashians' prior to her heavily publicised coming out as trans in 2015.

[6] Or at least trans people choosing to access medical services and present as male or female in a normative way, as Caitlyn Jenner typifies. Some individuals who strongly identify as non-binary may choose or desire to be read as binary some or all of the time (for example, Ash).

[7] Deadnaming refers to the practice of calling a trans person by the name they were given at birth, after they have taken a new name and asked to be referred to only by that name. For more detail of the political ramifications of deadnaming, see: http://fusion.net/story/144324/what-deadnaming-means-and-why-you-shouldnt-do-it-to-caitlyn-jenner/

[8] Be that 'treatment of a non-binary person' or 'medical interventions that do not follow a historically precedented masculine or feminine pathway'. The former has, fortunately, become more normalised in GICs as non-binary visibility has exploded within the last three years.

[9] In trans contexts generally, 'ffs' is an abbreviation of facial feminisation surgery. Here however, it stands for 'for fuck's sake'.

[10] Deeper critical context on this was given by Ruth Pearce in the conference paper 'Trans health research at a gender identity clinic', presented at the 2018 World Professional Association for Transgender Health (WPATH) biannual conference, in Buenos Aires. A recording and transcript of the paper are available here: https://ruthpearce.net/2018/12/18/clinical-research-with-trans-patients-a-critique/

[11] As there is no way to access the definitive purpose of questionnaire questions, this potential explanation is inevitably a speculation. However, it remains salient because of how trans service users engage in similar processes, in order to try and approach the questions 'correctly'. Indeed, Jamie suspected these questions to be connected to autism, and Simon Baron-Cohen's work on gendered brains specifically relates to a model of autism in terms of gender. Even if this is not the actual clinical usage of the question, it is how some patients interpreted it.

4

Non-binary times, non-binary places: communities and their intersections

> While community spaces can be seen to constrain queer subjectivities, then, queer identifications are also negotiated, vocalised and performed within community politics and locales. (Hines, 2010: 608)

Introduction

Time vitally intersects with non-binary identity negotiation across different forms of social interaction. Time spent introspecting can change self-conceptualisation, and time spent interacting with others can endear, or alienate. How an individual reacts to, interacts with, is affected by, or contributes to a particular community is dependent on the relationship an individual has with themselves. This changes over time, and may be shaped by communities, including those an individual is not a member of. Further, time is a critical and direct factor in particular circumstances that intersect with non-binary narratives, such as how long an individual may wait for a GIC appointment (see Pearce, 2018, chapter five), or how long an individual has benefited from (or lacked) community support.

Space is unavoidably connected to time in such contexts; for example, in cases where an individual's trans/non-binary status may be known in some settings but not others. The family home or the workplace may be spaces that restrict autonomy of expression, while queer community spaces may enable exploration.

While the title of this chapter was inspired by Halberstam's *In a Queer Time and Place* (2005), it otherwise does not directly build on postmodern, futurist work linking queerness with temporality (for example, Edelman, 2004; Muñoz, 2009). Rather, I draw attention to and unpack relationships with times and places that recur as sites of social significance for non-binary people, and the negotiation of identity. This builds on implicit references and crosslinks to time and place in Chapter 3, using time and space to collectively consider and connect aspects of lived experience through a sociological lens. This takes as axiomatic that the symbolic meanings ascribed to particular times and/or places are fundamentally informed by the interactions had within them.

I begin this chapter by considering how non-binary identities are negotiated over time, and how differences in subject positionality (particularly in relation to communities and medical practice) inform such a process. I explore participants' perspectives on the notion of non-binary identities potentially operating as a 'stepping stone' with which to explore gender, and from which some might then potentially 'arrive' at a binary-oriented trans identity. In such a case, one's status as non-binary may then be retrospectively positioned as transient, or liminal. The next section of this chapter then explores liminality in relation to non-binary (fittingly, sitting between the discussions oriented around time, and place). Importantly, it does not necessarily mean that non-binary identification is revised to having been 'less real' than a later identity. Rather, self-conceptualisation and comfort with gendering of the self may exhibit greater or lesser plasticity for different individuals, and the extent of this plasticity may change over time. Many participants recognised that non-binary can 'shift to binary' – and importantly, two of the participants (Jen and Frankie) specifically explained how this was true for them.

Conversely, participants also proposed that due to the lack of intelligibility of non-binary genders within some queer communities as well as wider society, binary-oriented trans identities may be 'found first' – particularly prior to an individual's involvement in communities that may expand their awareness of gendered possibilities. This can be part of a process that enables the development of, shift towards, or reinterpretation of gender in non-binary terms. Thus, non-binary identities may also be arrived at *following* a binary-oriented trans identification. This 'direction' of identity development (from binary to non-binary) was also experienced by some participants.

I then move to consider different contexts of 'place', though an analysis of community interaction discussed by participants. Some of these were not LGBTQ communities specifically, but other environments that created space to challenge gender norms or interact with gender in ways that participants felt helped them to explore being (or becoming) non-binary. This will conclude the 'community-oriented' pairing of Chapters 3 and 4, with Chapters 5 and 6 moving to the relationship between non-binary identities and clinical contexts.

Shifts over time: coming to identity through a 'stepping stone' process

Non-binary people's experiences of feeling delegitimised can be rooted in the problematic assumption that their identity is a phase. This perspective implies that non-binary people will, at some later point, identify within the binary as (trans or cis) men or women, and that consequently, non-binary identification is inherently 'unstable'. It bears a striking parallel to the disenfranchising pressure placed on bisexual people to 'pick a side', else be stigmatised as confused, greedy, indecisive or in denial (Callis, 2013).

Jess noted with some frustration how:

> 'I've met a lot of especially older trans women ... who have quite almost patronised me, come over to me and been like "Oh okay, well when you're ready to come to terms with being a trans woman, come to me and I'll help you navigate the process," or whatever. And quite often this is trans women who have actually been out as trans, navigating that system for a lot smaller amount of time than I have. So you know, I've been, I came out as genderqueer when I was 18, I'm now just coming up to 27, that's nine years of operating as trans and being out as trans. You suddenly have binary trans people who have been a couple of years into their transition leaning over and going "Oh come to me when you're ready," it's intensely patronising. So for a lot of the time it is seen as a stepping stone. And you know, actually, it can be a stepping stone. And there's nothing wrong with that.'
> (Jess, 26, interview)

Jess's feelings of being patronised are connected to having been out as trans for considerably longer than the women who offer their unsolicited advice and support. The trans women speaking to Jess implicitly position Jess's non-binary identity as transient or unstable, a product of 'not being ready to come to terms with being a trans woman', and liable to collapse as their presumed 'true' female identity emerges. Such communication functions as a microaggression (Chang and Chung, 2015), denying the validity of Jess's account of their non-binary identity as fixed/known (at least, as much as anyone else's). Further, there is an ironic sense of role reversal. The older individuals attempt to advise the younger; yet, Jess is more experienced, having been out for longer and being more experienced in navigating social interaction as transgender. Hence, Jess is older in terms of *trans time* (Pearce, 2019).

Jess's nine years out as genderqueer/non-binary provides a strong rebuff to claims of their identity being 'a phase', although this does not necessarily frame their gender as rigid. It is important to recognise how being non-binary does not need to be permanent in order to be respected. This is iterated through Jess's belief that the utilisation of temporary non-binary identification as part of a journey towards a binary (or more binary) subjectivity is not in itself a problem – "and there's nothing wrong with that" – such that non-binary people have no reason to feel threatened or undermined by those who previously identified as non-binary, but no longer do.

Pig's answer to the question 'Do you think people use non-binary identities as a stepping stone to binary identities?' was particularly interesting, because they firmly articulated the belief that it was "the opposite way around" – that is, some people use a binary-oriented trans identity as a stepping stone to a non-binary identity. Following this, I explicitly incorporated consideration of this position into future interviews, which yielded much support for Pig's claim.

> 'My colleague on the committee is post-transition for about a decade, probably a little bit more than that. He's fifty-odd. And he has told me on more than one occasion that had non-binary been an option, if he had known about it before he transitioned, he may not have transitioned, or he may have adopted this as his identity. And he's really not sure at all that he is a man, trans or otherwise post that transition. And I think that's an incredibly difficult position to be in after you have spent so much time and effort.' (David, 31, interview)

This example from David supports Jess's claim that some trans people who are positioned as 'detransitioning' might sometimes be better understood as coming into a non-binary experience of gender. Available, intelligible and 'respectable' transitions – social or medical – may be considered imperfect and uncomfortable by such individuals because they are highly constrained in binary terms, particularly historically. It's important to recognise that the negotiation of a non-binary identity cannot, in itself, be taken as indicative of a personal drive (or lack thereof) for medical interventions. That said, the binarised history of gender-affirming healthcare has meant that some of those who have felt an expectation to transition along a 'binary pathway' may not have done so (at least not in the same way), had an identity category and corresponding social possibility been available which didn't position hormones *and* genital surgery as necessary for the optimised, hegemonic trans subject.[1] I argue that this ultimately comes back to processes (and identities associated with them) that have been sheltered by the power of clinical legitimisation.

'I think that probably the majority of people who previously defined as binary who then go through a transition process to then detransition are actually non-binary, and they're not detransitioning to a binary gender which was the gender they were assigned at birth, but they are retransitioning to somewhere else. I think that if basically, if healthcare wasn't binary centred, we would be able to explore non-binary as an option and it not be seen as a stepping stone to binary people, but actually as a valid destination in and of itself.' (Jess, 26, interview)

Consideration of non-binary in relation to the concept of detransition has temporal ramifications. A simple reading of the detransition concept is strongly tied to regret: a notion of transition-as-mistake, and the assumption that anyone understood to be a detransitioner has a gender identity corresponding more or less with their assignment at birth. This discourse positions the symbolic totem of the detransitioner as a spectre of risk that haunts the clinician, and detransitioners themselves as tragic, mournfully wishing to turn back the clock, to unbecome. Non-binary is not an *essential* framework to conceptualise people renavigating medical or social transition in a manner different from this, but it does provide a clear motivational basis for 'detransition' (or rather, continued transition) that medical facilitators have historically neither embraced nor understood. Non-binary is therefore one of many sites where 'detransition' is not detransition at all, but a potentially positive process of temporal/embodied *re*-becoming.

Jess argues that it is important to provide space for the recognition of non-binary 'as a consistent state of being', but also acknowledges that gender identity can function in a transient manner. This deconstructs the further binary of permanence versus transience (Barker and Iantaffi, 2019), challenging the assumptions that permanence equals stability, and stability equals good mental health (and conversely, that transience means instability, and instability means being mentally unwell). The embeddedness of these assumptions can be seen in the context of pathways for medical transition and legal recognition in the UK, whereby trans individuals' 'change of gender role' is expected to be permanent and until death in order to be accepted as real, valid, and in *need* of gender-affirming medical procedures. This is due not only to the hegemonic presumption that gender identity is fixed across the lifecourse, but also to the traditional positioning of medical transition as the 'cure' for gender dysphoria, as associated with trans status.

In the case of David's friend, the apparent inability to articulate a non-binary identity was connected to *when* he negotiated gender transition, and correspondingly, his age. Trans time as a concept, then, does not speak solely to how long a person has understood themselves as trans; it also draws attention to how the *meaning* of trans will depend on when a transition happened and the concurrent community and medical discourses. We could consider a trans person at a point when they had been out for ten years. Being such was a radically different experience in 1979, 1999, 2019 – because of differently available discourses of gender, even having had the same amount of time to process, experience, grow and settle. Two people may be the same chronological age but have spent vastly different amounts of time aware of their transness and/or 'out' as trans. Conversely, individuals may have been out for the same amount of time but experience this very differently due to being different ages. Both forms of time will have significant impacts as to how a person relates to their own gender, and gender as an organising social concept (Pearce, 2019). The difficulty of renegotiating an identity after experiencing only a binary-gendered framework as possible for most of a lifetime may explain the finding from Harrison et al. (2012: 18) that 89 per cent of those identifying outside the gender binary were under the age of 45. Similarly, every member of this study was aged under 45 (Mark and Ricky were the oldest participants, both being 43 at the time). Moreover, the 11 per cent of non-binary people who *are* aged 45 or older are commonly neglected or erased in non-binary discourses, which in turn provides a limited number of possibility models[2] for other people of this age.

In contrast to the story of David's friend, the possibility of non-binary identification functioning as a transient step in negotiating binary identification is highlighted by the experiences of Jen and Frankie. Jen made contact via email after her interview, having reflected on the experience. Throughout her diary and interview Jen described herself as bigender, articulating that her self-expression (with regards to gendered presentation and desired embodiment) was dependent on whether she was in 'boy mode' or 'girl mode', but other aspects of her personality were not. In the email, Jen explained how the process of discussing identity and feelings regarding medical transition services through this project catalysed a process of introspective self-critique, which led her to the conclusion that she had been in denial over being a trans woman. Jen reconceptualised her experiences of fluidity as more accurately describing the extent of her dysphoria, rather than her gender at a given time. The significance of the correspondence necessitates its inclusion in full (with specific permission obtained from Jen):

Just want to say thanks again for the diary project and the interview. It's been really important for reflection. You were the first person to ask, in person, if I'd thought about HRT or surgery before. I'm sure I said something like "yes, I've thought about it, but I'd never do it" or something, but that conversation has had a big impact. Because you asked, out loud, I think it made me think differently about it. It's hard to explain but I guess I suddenly felt it was okay for it to be an option. Or I felt I was allowed to consider it. It's taken a long time to get from that conversation to here but I feel a lot clearer about several things. But I also feel kind of bad because in some ways I've been lying to myself, so that's reflected in my diary and interview.

Basically my description of sometimes feeling male and sometimes female is just not right and never has been. I think I've just told myself that so many times I kind of believe it. What's really fluid is how extreme the effects of dysphoria are (assuming I have gender dysphoria, I'm pretty sure I do but I haven't been diagnosed). What I call girl mode is me being female and having a really shit time with anxiety etc. what I call guy mode is me also being female but my mental health coping better. I still think of myself as female, I always want to transition, but because the dysphoria sort of comes in waves I can just keep my head down and get on with it. At first that meant pretending nothing was wrong. Then it meant coming out as non-binary. Then it meant describing myself as genderfluid so I could express myself but still have the option of "being normal" (yes I hate myself for that).

But really I've been asking myself the same question you asked me for months now and I feel like I've been in denial my whole life. I've gotten really good at telling myself I'm male. Anyway, I'm sorry if this messes up anything. I wasn't intentionally trying to deceive … it's more that I was lying to myself. I don't sometimes want to present as male and other times as female. I always want to present as female.

It's just I've learned to present as male to get on with it. So
if anything I'm presentation-fluid rather than genderfluid.
Or to simplify further, I'm a transwoman in denial. (Jen,
29, email)

I was humbled that Jen's involvement with this project assisted her in
renegotiating her identity in a manner she found to be illuminating.
The earlier text in Jen's diary was explicit in communicating that
non-binary fitted as an identity for her at that time. However, various
statements in the diary gain additional significance in the light of her
'confessional' email, such as "I'd love for people to see me the way I
feel, which is female," and "I don't feel I fit in as non-binary, or trans,
or bigender." This highlights how it is not only the passage of time
that has great potential to affect and enable gendered development, but
how one is engaged *during* that time: for example, with the research
interview providing a catalyst.

Jen recognises that non-binary identification was, for her, part of a
process of negotiating feelings of dysphoria, anxiety over not being
trans enough, and as she puts it, denial. These were significant factors
in constructing and constraining Jen's experience of her time as non-
binary (socially, and to herself). This also illustrates how the symbolic
meaning that one person associates with their identity can be quite
different from that of another, who experiences a different sense of
connection to the same term. That is to say: Jen's renegotiation of
identity and her relationship with gender cannot be taken as indicative
of others' experiences of bigender identification. The individual's
relationship with an identity category can easily transmute as factors
influence the relationship/fit between label and sense of self, over
time. This also demonstrates how the time participants spent reflecting
while producing diary entries was time that brought non-binary
into greater emphasis or focus (or scrutiny), with the interviews
serving to carve out and create additional time and space *for* non-
binary identities.

Identity shifts can also be tied directly to the progression of medical
transition, as described by Frankie:

Frankie: 'So, I think when I was writing the diary, I had a much
more kind of, my non-binary-ness was very apparent,
relatively apparent. I think when I was writing the diary
it was just at the start of kind of a bit of a shift? Which
I think is evident as I kind of go through to an extent.
But in the last few months I've become very grounded

in actually a more binary identity. A non-conforming female identity ultimately for me.'

Ben: 'I think you did start to say that, coming to the end of the diary. Do you still identify as non-binary?'

Frankie: 'To a small extent. I would call myself non-binary on occasion, but it's much, much less frequent than it used to be.'

B: 'Why do you think it is that you moved away from that?'

F: 'I'm really not sure. I think ... changes in my body? Definitely a catalyst. In terms of kind of feeling a bit more grounded in things.'

B: 'Do you think it gave you a sense of more ownership over inclusion in womanhood?'

F: 'Yeah, I think it did. I think kind of remapping my body ... yeah. In a way that I felt a lot more comfortable with than before.' (Frankie, 25, interview)

Access to hormones allowed Frankie to take ownership of an identity that resonated with their experiences of womanhood. In one sense, prior to medical intervention, Frankie's identity was constrained by feeling unable to claim being 'woman enough'. This demonstrates how medical discourses have shaped trans identity narratives, such that a lack of medicalised, embodied change can leave people feeling unable to claim transness or particular gendered identities that differ from the gender they were assigned at birth. Further, when Frankie says that they would call themself non-binary "on occasion", this implies that context may alter how one wishes to articulate one's gender identity, such that binary-oriented and non-binary identification are not necessarily mutually exclusive. This enables a reconceptualisation of the non-binary/binary binary(!) as instead, overlapping spaces. To be 'more' or 'less' binary is not to conceptualise male/masculine and female/feminine as two poles with a non-binary middle-ground, but is rather an entirely new axis of gendered consideration.

Figure 4 illustrates how a 'stepping stone' process of gender identification may be conceived. All individuals unavoidably have their earliest years constructed in relation to their assignment at birth. Those who are cisgender never (need to) question this assignment, even while great variations in terms of gendered conceptualisation, relationships with gender norms, presentation and behaviour exist within this 'box'. Those who come out as trans may articulate their identity in binary or non-binary terms, explicitly or not. How identity

Figure 4: Model of non-binary identity as a 'stepping stone' process

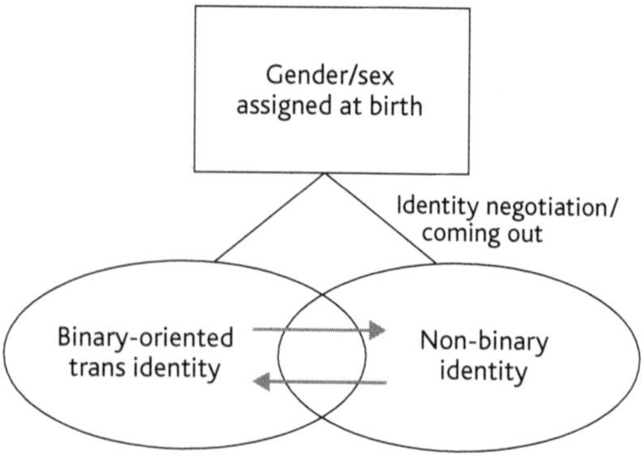

is articulated may also be dependent on factors such as time, space/ location/setting and social interactions. The large overlapping ovals signify fields within which an individual may be situated, such that different individuals may identify with the same generalising concept (within the gender binary, or not), yet still then experience or express gender very differently. The ovals overlap so as to signify the possibility of identification with binary-oriented and non-binary conceptions of gender simultaneously – such as identifying as a non-binary woman, as Jess did, and Frankie did also to a certain extent. The boundaries between the ovals should not be considered as fixed borders, but more equivalent to moving into/out of a patch of mist. One can know where one is situated and how to name where one is, but the boundary between is neither fixed, nor able to be straddled.

Jen and Frankie's narratives both follow the direction of the bottom arrow of the diagram, with initial negotiations of gender identity taking place within (very different) forms of non-binary conceptualisation, prior to continued negotiation that led to identification within the binary. While Jen positioned herself exclusively as woman, Frankie's description of themselves as non-binary in some situations allows their identity to be positioned within the overlapping section of the ovals, or on the edge of being/becoming 'only binary'. Other participants (such as Ash) negotiated both identity and transition in a binary-oriented manner, before revisiting changes to embodiment and social positionality years later, which would follow the trajectory of the top arrow in the diagram. A necessary caveat to this model is that it centralises a contemporary Western perspective. Being in a transitional state or at the boundaries of identity can be encapsulated by the concept of liminality, which is explored in the following section.

Betwixt and between: understanding 'in-betweenness' using the concept of liminality

The concept of liminality originated in the anthropological study of social rituals. It was used to describe the intermediate phase of a symbolically transformative process or transition, a Western example being baptism (Van Gennep, 1960). The concept was later expanded to address a wider range of transformative social processes that intersect with temporality, such as puberty (in-between adult and child), or war (in-between systems of stable rule). Relatedly, Monro (2007: 10) discusses how early transgender scholars 'describe transsexuality as a place outside duality'. The concept of liminality has been deployed in a wide range of sociological analyses of the 'in-between' that resonate with non-binary negotiations of queer communities and healthcare. These include representations of chronically ill or disabled people as neither 'sick' nor 'well' (Little et al., 1998), and accounts of identity reconstruction (Beech, 2011).

Liminality has been implicitly and explicitly deployed in transgender studies. In their work on the sociology of trans bodies, Ekins and King (1999) recognised narratives which 'transcend' the gender binary, creating practically infinite, fluid interpretations of gender that occupy a third category. Wilson has discussed the conceptualisation of liminal transgender identities, recognising the possibility that 'gender identities will not necessarily shift within this liminal phase, rather one's physical, behavioural and psychological self will be remodelled to "fit" with one's supposedly "transgressive" gender identities' (Wilson, 2002: 432). It is important to note while trans participants in Wilson's study identified as either transsexual or as cross-dressers, she 'found participants often grappling to identify themselves within the limited categories and scripts available to them' (Wilson, 2002: 431), which relates to the earlier discussion of possibility models and the temporally situated nature of becoming and being. Wilson additionally models trans community spaces as liminal, because they create possibilities for people who are not openly trans in their daily lives to become 'something else' for a limited time, specifically in that space. This understanding of community must be recognised as situated and partial. Community spaces may be experienced by many as sites where one can be oneself in a different way that is valued/enjoyed, but this needn't imply that one is not out as trans/non-binary in other contexts.

Connecting liminality and motion to narratives of gender transition, Carter (2013) discusses how in the historically significant Latin phrase *anima mulieris in corpore virilis inclusa* ('a woman's soul trapped in a man's body'), the word *inclusa*, which is translated to 'trapped' may instead be interpreted as 'enclosed', 'included', or otherwise allowing the possibility of motion rather than stasis. Medical transition is accordingly reconceptualised not in terms of *escaping* from the entrapment of the body, but instead in terms of the development and movement of identity over time, in relation to embodiment. This allows for movement in multiple directions, or motion backwards and forwards in a manner that defies hegemonic medical conceptualisation.

Both Frankie and Jen were clear that their past identification as non-binary was not viewed as a stepping stone or transient *at the time*. Non-binary was, for that period of their lives, the label they felt most accurately described themselves. Frankie said:

> 'It certainly didn't feel like [a stepping stone] consciously. Whether there was an element of that at a less conscious level is a debate, and I would say maybe there was an element. There's probably an element of truth in that. Whether people do that consciously or not, I think it's fine? Obviously. And you know, if people need certain identifiers and terms to be able to come to terms with their journey, more power to them for finding them and owning them at that point. I don't know, I would be surprised if anybody went into identifying as non-binary with a view that would then change, but maybe people do.' (Frankie, 25, interview)

Frankie's and Jen's experiences as non-binary can be understood as liminal, as this identification was for them an intermediary phase, positioned between (binary-oriented) identities. That Jen and Frankie contrast with Wilson's model of liminality (in renegotiating identity rather than forcing themselves to fit in) may reflect the great increase in access to a multiplicity of gender concepts, and moves towards their legitimisation by medical and community establishments. One critique of Wilson's frame is that it potentially implies an overly static, or essentialised, model of gender identity. That said, it's important to remember that trans/gender diverse discourses in 2019 are virtually unrecognisable compared to 2002; not only in terms of community size, heterogeneity and evolution of language, but also in terms of associated legislation.[3]

Support and validation from within trans communities can also fundamentally contribute to helping individuals feel like they can renegotiate how they wish to be understood. While not directly reflective of their experiences, both Jess and Frankie stated how consciously claiming an identity temporarily was entirely acceptable. Communities thus provide not only increased access to nuanced trans/gender discourses, but also the encouragement or security necessary to consider their relevance to one's own life, and acceptance that such relevance may be impermanent, without being of lesser validity or importance.

Liminality was of particular importance to Finn (22), who began their diary with this collage (Figure 5).

The dictionary definition of liminality which Finn provides implicitly positions the boundary in question as the gender binary,

Figure 5: Image of collage on liminality, from Finn's diary

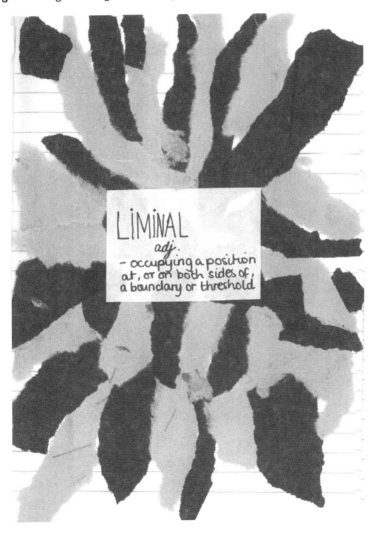

with clear symbolism in the surrounding tissue paper – shattered pieces of the classically gendered pink and blue. The central overlaid square box has neat, sharply defined edges, allowing for the interpretation that embracing a liminal state or identity that simultaneously occupies 'a position at, or on both sides of, a boundary or threshold' may grant stability. The chaos of gender remains outside of the box. While the coloured tissue is fractured and disorganised, it is notable that Finn did not include a third colour (such as purple). This fits with how non-binary presentation or embodiment may challenge a *demarcation* of what constitutes male and female (or masculine and feminine), yet struggles to be regarded as an intelligible category without reference to such constructed phenomena. Finn follows by discussing liminality, in saying:

> I don't see my identity or experiences reflected in either heteronormative or LGBT media ... I felt such a relief when I found the term 'non-binary'... but it also feels like I'm very much having to embrace my life as an 'other'. (Finn, 22, diary)

This highlights that the time of coming to, or 'arriving' at a satisfying identity cannot be simplistically viewed in only positive terms. There is a difference here to the 'classic' trans narrative where, for all the pain of dysphoria and stigma, encountering the concept of trans is discursively positioned as unshakeably and instantly recognised, and a straightforward degree of relief.[4] For binary-oriented and non-binary people alike, a non-cis gender modality (such as, but not limited to, trans) can be double-edged; catharsis may be found in intelligibility and sense making, but this is also associated with the risk of stigmatisation and violence.

A further example of liminal identity can be seen from Ash, in relation to embodiment. They said in their diary that 'I was particularly hoping to bleed this month so I could feel like a woman on National Women's Day ... But my body didn't co-operate and on National Women's Day I conceded it was an important day but not my day, not about me.' During the interview I followed up on this diary entry, to which Ash replied:

> 'I don't think [bleeding is] essential, I think if I really was a woman who was transgender or had a hysterectomy or whatever, I could totally accept that. But I think because I'm genderqueer, any sense of being a woman or a man is fleeting or unstable, and little things

my body does can make a difference to how I feel in a particular moment. I think that would've just pushed it over the edge and I would've felt a part of something even though I'm only in some way a woman and not in every way.' (Ash, 33, interview)

While Ash challenges the notion of biological essentialism in relation to claiming womanhood (Hale, 1996), it is nonetheless clear that physiological factors have an impact on their feelings about gendered embodiment, in conjunction with their fluidic, genderqueer identity. This connects back to how biological change through hormones and surgery can affect feelings of validity, as discussed in the previous chapter. Ash also acknowledges that their sense of being genderqueer can accommodate "fleeting and unstable" senses of being a woman, or a man. Ash's overarching non-binary identity can thus include situated feelings of maleness/manhood and/or femaleness/womanhood, which Figure 5 accommodates through the overlapping middle section. This particular example also highlights how diaries benefited the interviews, by allowing for the emergence of discussion points that I would not have incorporated into the topic guides had interviews been used alone.

While Ash is no longer undergoing any gender-affirming medical treatments (which historically would be associated with 'becoming' a man or a woman) their temporally specific experience in relation to National Women's Day relates their experience of gender to Finn's definition of liminality. Ash occupied a position at 'the threshold' of womanhood. The absence of bleeding prevented their self-conceptualisation as woman – not as a stand-alone phenomenon, but in the context of Ash's gender history. Such a discourse also opens the possibility of conceiving non-binary identification as a 'permanent liminality' – *constantly* in a state of becoming or flux, but without a static end point. Through the lens of liminality, then, non-binary gender identification can be conceived as a constant, unending process of 'becoming', but with moments or periods of particular impact. This is no 'more or less non-binary' than a fixed, stable sense of being neither man nor woman. However, it is also worth noting that due to the manner in which individuals change over time generally, and the centrality of gender to social interaction, the claim of 'an unending process of becoming' could also be applied to individuals regardless of gender identity, albeit so as to ignore the specific phenomenon of 'non-binary flux'. That is, for genderqueer or genderfluid individuals, the interactions that may directly play into experiences of gender shifting in day-to-day life – such as Ash's interactions with menstruation and

International Women's Day. Non- binary flux is intended to capture the ripples and shifts in gender identity among those who experience gender as fluidic, rather than 'renegotiations' of gender identity, such as coming out as trans/non-binary generally, or say, Jen's shift to a binary-oriented self-concept.

Charlie explored the concepts of non-binary flux and time using the outlet of poetry:

> I was woman
> once
> and woman I may be
> again
>
> but for now
> take me to the sea
> take my organs from me.
> take it all.
>
> And leave a tail
> and clamshell bra
> and give me power
> and let me swim.
>
> let me roam
> a world
> unruled
> by genitals (Charlie, 21, diary)

In positioning themselves as 'woman once', Charlie challenges the (sometimes strategically) essentialising 'born this way' narratives, used to demand respect and equal treatment *due* to gender being fixed and permanent in nature, which is discursively positioned as 'natural'. Likewise, they resist the normative pressure to position one's gender identity as *now* fixed, in acknowledging that they 'may be [woman] again'. There is ambiguity in the 'organs' Charlie refers to – while mastectomy is commonly associated with transmasculine identification and embodiment, elsewhere in their diary Charlie expressed a lack of desire for such a surgery, supported by the next verse in which they (still) wish for a clamshell bra. The organs could potentially be the uterus and ovaries; their connection to biological processes such as menstruation may, as with Ash, be connected to a sense of 'femaleness', though undesirably so in this context. Alternatively, 'organs' may be broadly symbolic of gendered embodiment; an interpretation supported by the line 'take it all'. This may be connected to the idea of death (and rebirth), where vital organs are taken (due to disease, or after death in order to be donated) to allow life, potentially disrupting the temporal binary of life and death as well as gender. In this context, being able to escape being positioned as 'woman' facilitates the articulation of a new life. The transformative theme of the poem may also be interpreted as a form of reincarnation – disrupting the binary and highlighting a liminal state between life and death.

The poem's ultimate focus is on recognising the distress and desire felt in a given moment, while recognising the possibility of future changes in desire. This raises questions about how time and liminality should be recognised within medical transition practices, as service users may need access to 'what is correct for them *now*', rather than 'correct' for them in an absolutist sense. The refusal or inability to perform 'certainty' regarding medicalised change and an associated projected future can position individuals as 'uncertain', making access to care more difficult. Should an individual articulate a fluid non-binary identity, and feel unable to definitively comment on future embodied desire or distress, this may result in a denial of currently desired treatment, even if the patient fully comprehends the significant and largely irreversible aspects of hormonal and/or surgical interventions. This is because 'uncertainty' (which may be assumed from any lack of presenting certainty) may inspire fear of the risk of regret, in an ultimately legally responsible clinician, and make them ambivalent or uncertain about providing access to treatment (Poteat et al., 2013). Such conservativism arguably runs counter to UK best practice guidelines which state 'patients are presumed, unless proven otherwise, capable of consenting to treatment' (Wylie et al., 2014: 169). The assumption that gender is a fixed and singular experience across the lifecourse deeply underscores current medical practice, such that narratives which resist this assumption may not be recognised as valid within medical or trans community settings.

Despite ultimately coming out as a woman, and renegotiating her prior bigender identity as indicative of 'denial' (or a liminal period), Jen articulated a point in her interview that may partially explain why she came out as non-binary first. She stated that, "it seems more extreme to come out as a trans woman". Thus, given her feelings of not fulfilling socially constructed criteria of womanhood *enough*, non-binary may have felt like a 'more reasonable' identity claim to make, when not (yet) possessing the 'legitimisation' of medical intervention. This can be seen in V's experience of identity negotiation in friends:

> 'Partly because of what I've said about the binaryness historically
> of the trans community, they've come out as non-binary first,
> and then when they've felt like their identity is legitimate enough
> in themselves, they've sort of ... transitioned to a binary, or
> started to use pronouns relating to a more binary gender. And
> literally only because of not feeling that they'd be accepted
> as trans if they turned up and didn't really hold to binaries.'
> (V, 28, interview)

V's account of the insecurities trans people can encounter through the fear that their experiences of gender variance are '[not] legitimate enough' relates to how an individual's sense of their own gender may change over time. Trans communities that reproduce or reify the gender binary as 'more' real, legitimate, or accepted (inadvertently or intentionally), will affect how individuals negotiate identity. This might lead people to reject non-binary identities on the basis that only a binary-oriented identity will be legitimised. Conversely, they may not allow themselves to adopt a binary-oriented trans identity if their community essentially sets up a gatekeeping logic whereby absolute certainty is necessary to be situated as 'binary trans'. The former is not to be confused with the additional possibility of individuals saying they are 'simply' trans men or women (while not identifying as such) to avoid delegitimisation. As Plummer (1995) articulates in his analysis of sexual stories, the possibilities of identity are modified by the social environments in which they are negotiated. Further, this is not to imply that the resultant binary identification arrived at by Jen and others is *inevitably* related to conscious or unconscious forms of social pressure. This is evidenced by individuals negotiating the reverse; in which a binary-oriented identity that was initially adopted through limited access to trans narratives, or through social pressure, is dis-identified with in favour of a non-binary identity.

There is a commonality between discourses of coming out as 'non-binary before binary', as V (indirectly, through accounts of friends), Frankie and Jen all articulate, and expressing identity as 'binary before non-binary', as Ash, Mark, and V (directly, discussing himself) did. Both involve the development of greater awareness of selfhood and gendered possibilities over time. This can occur through accessing community support, gaining awareness of new terms and language, building the confidence to re-declare one's identity, and/or resisting anxieties about being viewed as illegitimate. Such anxieties may involve not feeling trans enough to be binary, or positioning non-binary identification as necessarily unstable. As Alex put it in their interview, "I think people sort of view [non-binary] as a fake identity? You know, like a 'teenagers on Tumblr want to be different' identity." Here, non-binary is connected to adolescence, with both states positioned not only as liminal and unstable, but immature, in development, and a (temporary) phase. This shows how the gender binary can be positioned as so fundamental as to be unassailable, such that claims which destabilise it are relegated to ridiculousness, or assumed to be motivated by adolescent 'attention seeking'.

Some individuals may come out as having a binary-oriented identity rather than (or prior to) a non-binary identity because they perceive they will have greater difficulty being accepted, or in navigating gendered interactions, as non-binary. Although Jamie came out as non-binary, they did express some regret about having done so:

'The thing is, partly with me, it was a stepping stone. If I was coming out at work again now, I think I was really naive to think anyone would understand me when I said I'm non-binary and would actually treat me like I deserved any of the protections of the Equality Act. If I was coming out to people now, I'd say "I'm transgender" and only if they asked would I say I'm non-binary, and I would let people just assume I'm just the "opposite" of what I was assigned at birth. But I very much needed to go through a stage almost of saying "I'm not trans, I'm non-binary" because I didn't feel allowed to identify as trans, to get to the point where people identifying me as male socially is fine and makes me quite happy.' (Jamie, 24, interview)

There can consequently be a distance between how one wishes to (or does) identify in some spaces, and how one identifies personally, or in other spaces deemed to be safer and more supportive. This differs from strategic essentialism (Spivak, 1985) in that an epistemological primacy is not being utilised, though what Jamie wishes they had done may be conceived as 'strategic simplification'. In presenting themselves not as explicitly non-binary, but as transgender in an umbrella sense, Jamie would have relied on, by omission, people interpreting 'transgender' in binary terms, for the sake of social legitimacy and respect. Going into fuller detail for the sake of accuracy and honesty was felt by Jamie to only undermine their chances of being respected and legitimised, which relates to the comparative lack of cultural intelligibility and ontological validity of non-binary discourses. Interactions in different spaces can have particular significance for individuals, which I now move on to discuss.

Heterogeneity in community involvement

The relationship between being non-binary and the value of community is neatly introduced through David's discussion of how queer interaction affects their feelings about their identity. David articulated how the comfort provided by queer spaces affected their perception of what was 'normal':

> 'I've got a group of university friends who are currently having a WhatsApp conversation about us getting together, there are seven of us and I've just realised they're all straight! Everybody's going to be married very soon, and a couple of them have kids, and I'm like ... I'm not sure what to do with this, really! You're all so ... conventional!' (David, 31, interview)

Queer time and queer space are conceptualised by Halberstam (2005) as a framework for understanding queer experiences of difference, in relation to heteronormative practices of reproduction, marriage, and how they are timed and expected in relation to the lifecourse. David's sense of queer disconnect from the pressures and expectations of heteronormative family construction supports Halberstam's model of queer time, and highlights the importance of queer communities. However, David added that "you can't trust the LGB community to not be transphobic, because they quite blatantly are", highlighting the tensions that also exist in some queer spaces, with their accessibility partially dependent on the specifics of an individual's gender and sexuality.[5]

As discussed in Chapter 3, tensions can arise within trans communities through the policing of trans boundaries, such that some non-binary people feel excluded due to an anxiety of not being trans enough. LGBTQ community behaviours could also serve to alienate non-binary participants through more general problematic behaviours. After articulating discomfort with a university LGBTQ society, Alex explained this was due to some members:

> 'Just having very strong views which are not flexible, and you know, how I feel is that pretty much everyone's gender identity is unique, you can't say "this is how gender works" and then if people do say that, it annoys the heck out of me. And it also invalidates me when I'm different.' (Alex, 20, interview)

Leon illustrates how the binarised nature of community space wasn't necessarily produced (exclusively) by individual views, but the activities and discussions communities are oriented around:

'I'd been to FTM London [a trans support group] and I hated it; it didn't have any space for non-binary identities at all. I remember going to one meeting, and they had some people from Charing Cross talking, and it was packed out. A psychiatrist and an endocrinologist – and the endocrinologist was basically saying "You're all just men without testicles," and I was like "This is just *wrong*," and I left half way though and never went there again.' (Leon, 34, interview)

Leon's feelings about FTM London were not isolated. David, had also independently attended the group as a non-binary person not seeking medical transition. They felt that the group presented information in a way that assumed homogeneous interests and identifications among the membership:

'I worry that there might be people in the room going "Oh my god, I'm not interested in chest surgery, I'm not interested in hormones, why are you pushing me towards this?"' (David, 31, interview)

Further to specific concerns related to non-binary identification, Leon and David also discussed experiences with queer communities which did not recognise any trans/non-binary people. David discussed in detail the negotiations with the LGB group at their place of work, highlighting how the conspicuous absence of the 'T' in the abbreviation positioned them as both out of touch and failing to offer an inclusive space. Leon explained how, when trying to work with an LGBT swimming group, they were told 'we don't have any trans people'. The fact that the swimming group positioned itself as LGBT, yet, both in their interactions with Leon and in their club information, only discussed the possibility of gay men and lesbian women being members, illustrates how the presence of the 'T' cannot be taken to assume awareness and inclusion of transgender people. Dean Spade (2004: 53) has dubbed this exclusion, through the collapse of LGBT into 'sexuality only', as 'LGB fake-T'. Despite not necessarily requiring specific policies in the same way that trans people may, this association of LGBT exclusively with gay men and lesbian women is also an example of bi-erasure (Barker and Langdridge, 2008).

David recognised the problem of interactions being derailed by basic issues of transgender (though particularly non-binary) recognition and respect, through a fictional conversation recorded in their diary:

> "Isn't it a beautiful day today? I hope X enjoys it, she is always saying how much she loves the sunshine"
>
> "Actually, X uses the pronouns "they/them/their". But it is a very beautiful …
>
> "Oh God I am so sorry, it's just so difficult for me. But now that we are talking about this, can I ask you about gendered pronouns? What's a pronoun anyway? How can 'they' be singular? [...]
>
> Etc. etc. ad nauseam and, in the meanwhile, the beautiful day has been forgotten and the day is all about pronouns now. (David, 31, diary)

This allegory by David can be used to understand the potential educational and emotional labour (Martínez-Iñigo et al., 2007) that may be expected from people as a direct consequence of their being openly non-binary. Emotional labour is associated with how feelings need to be managed and expressed as part of particular paid employment roles (Hochschild, 2012). 'Bedside manner' has been studied as an example of emotional labour in clinical contexts (Larson and Yao, 2005), but I argue that emotional labour can usefully capture the emotional and communicative regulation that gender-diverse people can perform when interacting with clinicians (or other holders of authority) in order to fulfil an aim – such as accessing a referral or a diagnosis. This can also be felt within mundane social contexts (for example, interactions with non-queer people and the micro-interactions associated with, for example, shopping). However, it is significant that in queer communities, too, non-binary people cannot necessarily find a space or time in which they might hope to presume they will be intelligible or met with respect.

Multiple participants specifically mentioned cisgender gay men as a particular source of tension or intolerance in queer communities. Hal said:

> 'With the queer community, gay men, they can be really dismissive. You go from straight guys who are just being "Oh that's queer," to those who say "Oh that queen is giving us all a bad name. Why can't you keep it together and be normal like the rest of us?" ... I get it most from guys who call themselves

'straight acting', their masculinity is very important, and they don't like people saying deviation is perceived as part of the same group.' (Hal, 42, interview)

The pressure to 'be normal like the rest of us' speaks to a respectability politics produced through an assimilatory homonormativity (and cisnormativity) that may be found among some LGBT people, to the detriment of those positioned as most (visibly) transgressive (Duggan, 2002). Charlie and Frankie give further particular examples of behaviours and responses to their gender identities they especially associated with cis gay men:

Charlie: 'I see some of it [people policing others in queer communities], especially in the university LGBTQIAA+ society. I don't especially like to be a part of that group of people because whilst some of them are really great, with such a wide and varied group of people there will be people with some negative opinions of non-binary people, or people that if they're non-binary they're not subverting the binary enough, they feel.'

B: 'Do you see that sort of negativity coming from particular demographics at all?'

C: 'Yeah. It's often ... some of it's been a lot of cisgender white gay men. But also there are transgender people who are more binary in the group who say things like that, and yeah.' (Charlie, 21, interview)

Ben: 'Have you ever had experiences where your identity is being challenged or invalidated by other queer people?'

Frankie: 'Yeah. I think assumptions have definitely been made, I think in the past when I used queer as a term to describe myself, the assumption was made that I was a cis gay male. And people thought I was talking about being interested in men, and it very much came from a sexuality assumption, looking through a very cisnormative lens.'

B: 'What sorts of people were making that assumption?'

F: 'Mostly cis gay men? [laughs] To be honest, but occasionally others as well. Usually always ... I say usually always cis people, but some trans people as well.' (Frankie, 25, interview)

In these examples, different responses to non-binary people within queer spaces could function to cause tensions. For Hal, who discussed experiencing being mistaken as a gay man exhibiting femininity, gay men whose sensibilities are informed by homonormative values could stigmatise them. This is explained through Stryker's analysis that gay and lesbian assimilation may be threatened by non-normative trans articulations and needs (Stryker, 2008b).

The cultural dominance of gay men within many LGBTQ spaces may also help explain why despite its deliberate and subversive ambiguity, the subtext of certain queer spaces may assume a 'sexuality exclusive' reading of queer. This runs contrary to an active recognition and inclusion of gender-diverse people, even while drag artistry is often embraced. We also see from Charlie that through a lack of cultural intelligibility or through transphobia, cisgender members of queer communities are by no means necessarily recognising or supportive of non-binary people. Charlie also raised the possibility of non-binary people being challenged for 'not subverting the binary enough'. This relates to Mark and V's discussions in Chapter 3, where it was recognised how some individuals could challenge the authenticity of others in order to gain a hierarchical sense of self-validation. As non-binary awareness increases, so does the chance of stereotypes being propagated, and non-binary people being held to these as yardsticks of authenticity. With non-binary identities sometimes positioned as particularly 'subversive', it is worth recognising how non-binary people may also engage in such negative practices to other non-binary people.

While cis men were highlighted more frequently than any other demographic, Ricky discussed coming out as non-binary in the context of a lesbian community:

> 'There was a lot of ... "How are you different from me?" with lesbian friends. A lot of competitive stuff as well, of like, you know "Well I identify as a woman, but I'm way more masculine than you, so how dare you identify as something nearer male than I do!"' (Ricky, 43, interview)

This illustrates that some LGBTQ people (such as the butch lesbians Ricky is referencing) may problematically construct their sense of validity of masculinity or femininity in a comparative, competitive and oppositional manner to other community members. Additionally, 'masculinity' and 'maleness' may be conflated, such that AFAB individuals who are not particularly masculine claiming a non-binary identity may anger or offend masculine, butch women for whom being assigned female corresponds with their self-conceptualisation. Some members of lesbian communities have argued that lesbian identity formation can be disrupted by queer and trans discourses, as may the ability of lesbian communities to produce effective social activism (Shugar, 1999). Such tensions along boundaries of identification may feed into non-binary people's sense of insecurity over being trans enough, or in the context Ricky raises, not masculine enough to 'enter into' transness – reminiscent of the earlier 'butch/FTM border wars' (Halberstam, 1998). The affronted response of some butch lesbians was a result of their perception of dissonance between Ricky's identity and the butch lesbians' expectations of masculinity and femininity in relation to gender identity. With butch lesbians articulating masculinity but without rejecting femaleness, there was a sense that non-binary people (being situated as 'less female' than them) 'need' to be correspondingly more masculine. From the butch lesbians' perspectives, Ricky failed to be adequately masculine to claim non-binary, and was viewed negatively as a consequence. This approach continues to situate AFAB experiences of non-binary identities as an incomplete, partial, or lesser trans masculinity, rather than as a state of being that does not exist in a hierarchical relationship with binary-oriented trans identification. The rationale holds when considering AMAB individuals (who may be situated as an incomplete, partial or lesser trans femininity), but there isn't a clear parallel of community politics between AMAB non-binary people and feminine gay men.

It is, however, important to emphasise that this collection of experiences does not reflect a universal dissatisfaction with LGBTQ spaces for non-binary people. Rather, they highlight that navigating non-binary experience in queer communities can cause difficulty or alienation, through the cultural unintelligibility or perceived tensions caused by non-binary extending well into some queer spaces, rendering them uncomfortable, or creating obstacles for inclusion, understanding and/or respect. Further, the manifestation of this tension can depend on the specific context, such as whether it is a generalised LGBTQ space, or one with a more specific target demographic (be that age, as in most student groups, or gender/sexuality intersection, as in lesbian groups).

In addition to discussing experiences of queer communities where 'queer' has been broadly synonymous with (any part of) LGBT, multiple participants used the potential broadness of 'queer' to discuss experiences of communities beyond LGBTQ – conceptualising spaces as queer that are not inherently focused on gender and sexuality minority identities. This also raised the significance of additional community groups for non-binary identity negotiation.

Within kink communities, the importance of consent both in and beyond sexual activity is positioned as an essential community norm (Barker, 2013a). Alex illustrated how consent culture[6] (Barker, 2013b) had positive ramifications for their feelings of validation and respect regarding their gender:

> 'When I was kind of struggling with my gender identity a bit, someone referred to me as a lady at a kink event, and I said "I'm not a lady, I'm a barbarian." And there were some people, who, because they didn't know if I was serious or not, they referred to me as a barbarian ever since. [...] They were willing to do that, even though I was just kind of being stupid ... That's amazing. I love getting that sort of thing from people. People are obviously much less questioning of things like clothing choices in that community.' (Alex, 20, interview)

Despite speaking favourably of the kink community, Alex also told an anecdote in which everyone attending a particular event was asked to write their name down on a piece of paper that had separate 'male/female' columns; consequently "a bunch of us wrote our names down the middle, and then they stopped doing it". Alex also drew attention to kink events failing to take any action in relation to male and female toilets being the only available options (such as creating temporary labels to indicate gender-neutral bathrooms). Further, Alex articulated that they felt the dress code of the kink group they engaged with was transphobic "because it's got to be kink wear, and kink wear is very different for female or male bodies". Despite it being entirely permissible for an AMAB person to wear fishnets and heels, for example, they explain:

Alex: 'The men have to wear formal clothing. But then I just wander around in tracksuit bottoms and I can get away with it because I get my tits out. And I don't think that's okay. I don't mind because I want to wear suit trousers but I don't think that should be a rule.'

Ben: 'So, for example, a trans woman couldn't wear the bottoms that you'd want because of how they'd be read?'

A: 'Yeah.' (Alex, 20, interview)

The point Alex is making is that while the group has rules that a particular level of formality is required, those individuals with breasts can easily ignore such rules for the clothing on the lower half of their bodies, precisely because of their breasts, which Alex positions as unfair. Thus, the symbolic reading of the bodies of trans people may result in being treated differently (in a manner that delegitimises their genders) from cis bodies. This would likely be dependent on transition or point of transition – the trans woman without breasts having her experience differentiated from the trans woman (or cis woman, or pre- or non-operative AFAB trans person) who has. The non-binary or transmasculine body with breasts is thus also positioned as female by the community's cisnormative perceptions of bodies in clothing associated with kink. This links back to how trans bodies which have received medical interventions are more likely to allow for identity to be respected and positioned as '(more) real'.

Relatedly, Bobby discussed their involvement with the Lolita community.[7] The openness towards different gender identities in Lolita space allowed individuals to explore their relationship with femininity through a hyperfeminine-oriented style and subculture. Bobby illustrated this style in Figure 6.

> 'There's a load of "Brolitas" which is like cis male Lolitas that have all of the dress and the bows and fells and usually have a wig. I think a lot of people go through the stages of working out where they are on the [gender] spectrum, by going out one stage at a time like "I am a cis person, but I am just going to wear this item of clothing," and "Oh I'm not sure anymore, maybe I am a non-binary person or whatever."' (Bobby, 23, interview)

Bobby's drawing was included in their diary in part as a conscious effort to ensure that I (the researcher/reader) would comprehend the community being discussed. This serves to reiterate that participants, to greater or lesser extents, constrained or structured their diary entries on the basis of their perceptions or assumptions regarding my knowledge or views. Material was sometimes crossed out or corrected, with the starkest confrontation being in Ash's diary, who wrote 'Who are you Ben Vincent, what does your diary contain? You know lots about me if you've read this far. I know less about you. I wonder what you think of me. Like me. Like me. Please like me.'[8] This was followed by a reflection on the 'instant reward' of social media use, highlighting the temporal dimensionality of diary keeping – in which revisiting what was written in different contexts and for different reasons may catalyse valuable new formulations. Bobby's Lolita community differed from an LGBT-specific community, in that involvement in the former

Figure 6: Sketch showing Lolita fashion, from Bobby's diary

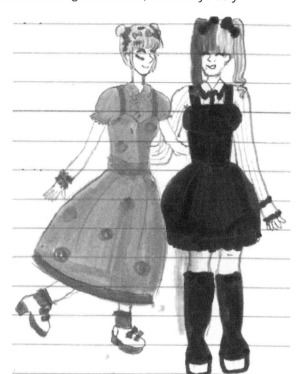

did not imply any particular relationship with sexuality or gender identity. Yet, it still provided a space for gendered exploration – indeed, a form of exploration not specifically possible in an LGBTQ setting, due to the differences between constructing a 'Lolita look' and wearing drag. In being structured exclusively around style, the Lolita group produces different discourses from 'crossdressing' in specifically LGBTQ community contexts.

Both Ricky and Ash highlighted their positive experiences with bi communities. Ash shared the view that "most, if not all" people in bisexual communities were aware of and friendly towards trans/non-binary people. In explaining what it was about bi communities that made them more "ambiguity positive", Ricky explained:

'I think for a start that once if you recognise that you're attracted to more than one gender then I guess you're possibly more open to the idea that there isn't this "there are two genders and they're the complete opposite of each other and never the twain shall meet" – I think that's part of it. I think the bisexual community is much more open to the idea of fluidity and flexibility and ambiguity, whereas hetero and gay spaces tend to be, you're either one thing or the other.' (Ricky, 43, interview)

Bisexual identification has a history of being relegated to a temporary state ('you are just not sure') or an immoral one ('you are being greedy', 'bisexual people will cheat') both within and outside queer communities (Alarie and Gaudet, 2013; Monro, 2015). It is intuitive, then, that a sense of recognition and solidarity might be seen between individuals breaching the gay/straight binary of sexuality and the male/female binary of gender. Importantly, bisexual community spaces are also changing over time in direct response to voices and forms of resistance within them. Ash gave the example of how the intersection of gender identity, race and sexuality has been addressed at an annual bisexuality convention:

'An example was at bi-con. I went to one of the workshops ... there was exclusive spaces for trans people of colour, and those people came together ... and they started to talk about the ways they experienced racism in bi-con specifically. And then they started to send somebody out to liaise with the organisers, talking about ways to make it better. Trying to educate some people about how to be better and more respectful, and actually what they were talking about this year was the great extent to which that's been achieved now, and people are coming into the space not with an awful lot of grievances that need correcting but generally quite happy with the space. So just talking how that's good, and how useful it was to have that exclusive space and come together with people who understand, talk about the problems, and when they've got something coherent they want to ask for, come to the rest of bi-con and ask for it. So that's an example how that space was rubbish but has improved.' (Ash, 33, interview)

This example exemplifies how, within a time/space for queer community, a demarcated area amplifying more marginalised voices and engaging with intersectional inequalities might serve to address wider issues. The similarities and differences between the struggles of the civil rights movement and of LGBT liberation have been compared in a legal context, in terms of what the latter can learn from the former. One of the central points of import in this analysis was how LGBT rights groups must 'take care not to exclude, either by acts of commission or omission, people at the fringes of the movement' (Neal, 1995: 681). While it would be a mistake to assume that non-binary people are 'at the fringes' of queer communities due to their relatively recent increase in recognition, Ash's example does show how sincere and significant efforts by organisers to create space for marginalised voices can serve to improve the community's reputation more generally. Community practices in particular spaces, or at particular times, can thus bring greater particularity to members' needs (Hines, 2006).

Conclusion

In this chapter I first focused on how binary-oriented and non-binary (trans) identities can each function to lead to the other, and how this may be catalysed through embodied personal desires connected to medical transition. This was related to negotiations of the self over time, such that the experience of being binary or non-binary can be understood as liminal – that is, either existing on two sides of a boundary at once, or occupying a fluid, evolving, transitional middle point in a social process.

I then explored how participants *viewed* non-binary identities as a stepping stone to binary identities, and vice versa. Participants gave varied accounts and explanations which showed how both scenarios occur among trans/non-binary populations, while also demonstrating the possibility of identifying simultaneously with and outside the gender binary. I constructed a model to illustrate how understanding the movement of identity over time is important to gain a nuanced understanding of individuals. This also emphasises how 'trans' can involve the transition not only of the body – as emphasised in medical literature – but also of identity through and over time, which incorporates how one is socially interpreted and interacted with – a challenge to any universalisation of the 'X trapped in a Y's body' narrative. The story of trans self-negotiation in relation to gendered expectations has historically been told in a manner that focuses on embodiment and surgery, which has had notable and tangible effects even for those who are not attempting to access medical intervention, but who simply seek social recognition, validation and equal treatment.

Likewise, I have explored the ways in which community spaces are needed, and touched on how some of these have changed over time. Difficulties or tensions can be created through the binarised or medicalised focus of some lesbian, gay, bisexual, trans and/or queer communities, the potential for off-putting, non-inclusive views among some members, plus the existence of names, official information or practices that erase trans or non-binary lives. However, community groups that are not trans focused, or even necessarily LGBTQ focused, can be of great importance and benefit to non-binary people, and demonstrate reflexive and intersectional practices of inclusion. Diverse communities that are 'gender-adjacent' (that is, with ramifications around gender expression but not centred on gender per se) such as kink or Lolita scenes are under-researched in relation to trans/non-binary experiences – though recent work by Pearce and Lohman (2019) has considered transness in relation to alternative music scenes.

I conclude that regardless whether individuals experience non-binary identity as liminal, fluid or static, it is useful to consider identity formation as a temporal process which has no fixed end. Many of the positive and negative experiences that different participants reported were linked to particularities of space, and who occupies the space – often informing the levels of sensitivity and knowledge that could be expected during interactions. Further, as time passes, individuals are able to adjust, explore and become comfortable with these important factors relating to non-binary experience. This chapter has also served as a foundation for the consideration of non-binary clinical interactions in the following chapters, as both individual and community-oriented experiences over significant lengths of time are deeply significant for understanding trans healthcare.

Notes

[1] I do not make any assumption about the medical interventions that David's colleague has accessed, as the argument does not ultimately depend on this. In short, we are looking at the temporal dimension of the problematic notion of 'more medical interventions equal a firmer ontological claim on one's gender (and gender modality) when trans'. The most classic cisgenderist example of this might be the view that achieving 'real' womanhood/manhood *depends* on accessing vaginoplasty/phalloplasty.

[2] This conceptual reframing as an alternative to 'role models' has been pioneered by Laverne Cox. See: www.radiotimes.com/news/2015-07-26/orange-is-the-new-blacks-wonder-woman-laverne-cox-on-being-a-transgender-trailblazer/

[3] Key examples in the UK being the full repeal of section 28 (of the Local Government Act 1988), in 2003, and the creation of the Gender Recognition Act 2004 and the Equality Act 2010.

[4] Of course, this is not true for many binary-oriented trans people, who may take years or decades to process their relationships with gender prior to coming out. However, 'knowing that one was different' from a very early age, and 'bolt of lightning' recognition remain staple elements of classical expectations of trans being and trans becoming (see Kennedy, 2019).

[5] This also raises the point that many LGBT spaces, such as clubs, bars or saunas, may be very (cis) male dominated/oriented, and not particularly welcoming for cis lesbians or bisexual women, in addition to the dimensionality of trans awareness.

6   Whereby consent does not exclusively operate at the level of individual, interpersonal interaction, but is embedded across the community such that responsibility for ethical practices and avoidance of harm is shared.

7   In this context, a Lolita is an individual involved with the Lolita fashion subculture, which originated in Japan. The community is centred on the construction of modest, hyperfeminine, identifiably stylised garments to create a 'Lolita look'.

8   The first time I read this moved me to tears, underscoring the significant emotional impact that research enterprises can have on participants and researchers, and the ethical responsibilities these entail, including to ourselves (see Dickson-Swift et al., 2009).

5

Views of the clinic: non-binary perceptions and experiences of general healthcare services

Those who identify 'beside' the gender binary will still be situated within it by others whose worldviews are bounded by the discourse of binary gender, such that it is impossible to escape this discursive framework altogether. (Sanger, 2008: 50)

Introduction

This and the following chapter will focus on non-binary perceptions of healthcare in the UK. In this chapter, I address primary care services for the most part (with some mention of secondary care), focusing on both the views and experiences participants reported of interactions with doctors and other staff, such as nurses and administrators. Secondary care practitioners whose fields are unrelated to gender transition will have, on average, similar knowledge of trans healthcare needs as primary care practitioners. Such discussions are addressed within this chapter. Further, the motivation for a non-binary service user to access secondary care may be very broad, the same as with cisgender service users. This is not the case when a secondary care service has been accessed, for example, on the advice or referral from a gender identity clinic (GIC). Secondary care services that are routinely used as a consequence of GIC access (such as some endocrinologists and psychiatrists) will have experience and approaches in closer alignment to tertiary care gender specialists. Therefore, these medical experiences are addressed in Chapter 6.

I begin this chapter by considering how participants judged the non-binary community's overall view of care when going to a GP. This is followed by specific accounts and examples of individual's experiences of primary care, for appointments not related to gender transition. This begins with experiences of 'gendered medicine' – healthcare which is differentiated in gendered terms, such as smear tests. This is followed by generalisable healthcare experiences, such as arm pain. Some experiences resonate strongly with binary-oriented trans experiences of primary care (Feldman and Goldberg, 2006; Dewey, 2008). Responses from doctors to patients that may be ideal for a binary-oriented trans person may or may not work for a non-binary patient. Some participants discussed positive views of general medical practice, while simultaneously reporting an overall negative and guarded sense regarding medical practice in gender-diverse communities.

This leads to an important sub-group of clinical experiences, those non-binary people who also experience chronic illness and disability, and the interplay between these experiences. Finally, this chapter addresses how clerical administration in medical institutions may affect non-binary patients. This includes discussion of how names and pronouns are used and recorded, and medical forms specifically discussed by participants – including feedback forms and documentation related to tertiary care. While this chapter is structured around primary care, the cross-practice nature of administration renders a general discussion that cuts across all forms of care appropriate. Discussion of the key administrative process of referral brings this chapter to a close. This section also serves to link to the following chapter on GIC care, much as the referral acts to bridge from the GP to GICs within practices of care.

Non-binary views of primary care

Some participants communicated views of primary care that were overall impressions, rather than linked to specific experiences. Some made it clear that positive (unspecified) experiences shaped their view.

> My experience has been overarchingly positive in terms of the NHS. Medical staff seem concerned with functionality, and unconcerned with social labels. True, not so long ago medical systems couldn't cope with assigning a male pronoun to a patient owning a vagina. However, this is different now. (V, 28, diary)

V was keen to highlight how differences could be seen between the present and the recent past, emphasising the importance of how changes over time in medical practice influence an individual's views. Observing 'medical systems' changing first-hand may reshape the extent of an individual's confidence in practitioners regarding trans cultural competence. Frankie had positive and negative feedback to share, but reported their belief that other people's experiences tended to be negative:

'[Trans people's experiences of medical practice are] not good! Generally not good. That said, you don't normally hear people being particularly vocal about the good experiences they've had. The ones you do hear about tend to be the negative ones ... Yeah, just a lot of misunderstanding, a lot of barriers put up to medical assistance. Accessing things that need to be accessed, or that have been accessed for a long time but because someone's changed their circumstances, moved GP or something, they have to go through a whole lengthy process again just to get their prescription moved, and this that and the other. So yeah, generally not good, but then that might be kind of slightly tainted by the fact that I work in wellbeing, work with trans people, generally have to deal with difficulties rather than positive experiences.' (Frankie, 25, interview)

Frankie recognises the possibility of being exposed to particularly negative views of medical care through working with trans people accessing support. This recognition may have potentially been nucleated by these negative accounts clashing with their own broadly positive experiences. When asked their thoughts on the medical establishment's interactions with non-binary people, Alex said:

'I think it's very bad at recognising them. There's a lot of misgendering. I've had quite good experiences with that personally, but I know there is a lot of people who report being misgendered, who report having poor interactions with the medical establishment based on that.' (Alex, 20, interview)

This reiterates the theme that even when having positive experiences personally, participants did not then dismiss or play down what they heard through community networks of other people's negative experiences. Therefore, the relative impact of negative experiences on an individual's conception of medical service provision is higher. Relatedly, it has been found that individuals who associated or experienced stigmatising behaviour from healthcare practitioners anticipated this more generally (Earnshaw and Quinn, 2012), implying that negative experiences will have a deeper impact on views within a community than positive experiences. This will be considered in more detail in relation to gender transition-oriented care in Chapter 6.

One specific critical view of primary care practitioners that was aired by multiple participants was the tendency for other medical conditions or diagnoses to be ignored in trans individuals, instead connecting unrelated complaints to gender identity. Some participants highlighted this through a comedic yet exasperated tone:

> Got acne? It's because you're trans*[1]
> Aching muscles? It's because you're trans*
> Headaches? It's because you're trans*
> Bruised toe? Because you're trans*
> Stress? Trans*
> Trans*
> Trans*
> Trans* (Mark, 43, diary)

> 'I didn't have good experiences with doctors at uni[versity] at all. They don't ever believe anything's wrong with you, they just think you're stressed. Or at least my doctor it was always "are you feeling stressed, are you getting enough sleep, are you eating enough", it's what people say about being trans; you've got a trans broken leg!' (Jamie, 24, interview)

Further, Jess gave evidence to the Women and Equalities Committee[2] held by the government on 8 September 2015. She stated:

> We call it the trans cold. If you go to your doctors with a cold it will be a trans cold. Quite literally, my housemate has had a throat problem for the last year or so and has been taken to Ear Nose and Throat, and the doctor diagnosed her with 'transgender problems', that's literally the words he wrote on the piece of paper. (Women and Equalities Committee, 2015: time stamp 11.52.08)

These incidences serve to highlight the sense within trans communities that primary care practitioners may articulate an inappropriate fascination with an individual's trans/non-binary status, which may hinder access to appropriate medical care for health issues unrelated to trans status. The potential fear of voyeuristic attitudes from primary care practitioners regarding transgender status risks alienating some individuals from accessing healthcare in a timely manner (King, 2016).

In addition to descriptions and discussions of how experiences of primary care related to their genders, some participants talked about how they felt alienated from their GPs because of the impression they received of them more generally. Participants could extrapolate their concerns, such that they felt there was an unacceptable level of risk regarding communicating being non-binary with their GPs.

Hal went into detail when relating how they felt they should make an appointment to discuss ADHD (attention deficit hyperactivity disorder) medication, but had misgivings:

> I realised it's not just the stress and workload that is keeping me from booking an appointment with my doctor. It is also the fact that he is very conservative ... His nurses and staff also make me uneasy. Uneasy enough that I have to prepare myself mentally before I go to the clinic; make sure that there are no traces of nail polish or mascara visible on me and dress carefully in what I call my "office drag". It doesn't make me feel good. It actually feels awful to be so afraid of these people judging me at a moment when I feel pretty vulnerable already. I should get another GP. (Hal, 42, diary)

By 'office drag', Hal is referring to a normative, masculine appearance in order to 'pass' as cisgender. Articulating this as drag indicates Hal's sense that this presentation is affected and performed, as a protection against potential stigma in this context. Hal connected the Conservative political affiliation of his physician with a morality and worldview that made them "afraid of these people judging me". Fear of stigma when already feeling vulnerable had a significant impact on Hal's willingness to attend the doctor's at all, which compounded the stress and workload they initially mentioned, to render primary care considerably less accessible. Frankie had a similar experience:

> 'My GP made a big point of being like "We don't know anything about this, we're a very conservative community," as if that somehow meant that they didn't need to know about it.' (Frankie, 25, interview)

Frankie's GP also made demands of them to "explain what being a trans person is", emphasising the unrecognised educational and emotional labour that can be demanded of trans patients; that is, gender-diverse patients may need not only to unpack a conceptualisation of gender identity for a provider when access to appropriate support may be contingent on their understanding, but also to perform geniality as part of massaging the doctor-patient interaction. Jess expressed the same anxiety as Hal, having not seen a "doctor, or a dentist, or a medical health professional of any kind" in the nine years since she came out as non-binary. Jess explained this in relation to multiple overlapping loci of negative medical associations. First, she explained how she felt if she went to the doctor's she would "have to start that conversation about gender" which could "rope [me] into a binary transition pathway which I'm not sure I want". This concern expresses an anxiety with potential lack of agency in the doctor/patient interaction (Newman and Vidler, 2006). Jess and Hal's feelings illustrate a sensitivity, both to the views that doctors (may) hold as well as the view, or clinical gaze (Singer, 2006) exerted over the non-binary body.[3]

Second, Jess's activist work of training doctors in trans healthcare means that they "see it behind the scenes", and are apprehensive to receive insensitive or substandard care due to being non-binary. Like Frankie, Jess is exposed to a great deal of negative narrative, but without the mitigating positive personal experiences Frankie recounted. Finally, Jess alluded to negative experiences as a disabled child accessing medical care for their impairment, highlighting how intersections with chronic health conditions and disability concerns must be recognised when considering trans/non-binary health.

As Jess and Frankie's accounts have alluded, it is important to recognise that not all perceptions of primary care experienced by non-binary people will be from the position of being a patient. Alex discussed their experiences as a student nurse, and working in healthcare as a non-binary person in their diary. In particular, they discussed that a department they worked in made an accusation of them relating problematically with others, which was sent to their academic tutor. These were not acted on, but Alex articulated how they were positioned as being uncommunicative and not engaging in their departmental handover process. Alex explained their belief that this was due to how they interacted with their nursing colleagues/instructors socially, rather than professionally. It was Alex's view that due to being positioned as/ assumed to be female, they were accordingly held to gendered social norms. When not offering expected cues in response to "conversation about celebrities, when they all talked about 'being good' and watching what they ate", Alex viewed this to be the reason they were judged negatively, despite holding that "by male standards I was fine; it's just unusual for 'women' to not conform to certain behaviours".

This account highlights the gendered nature of the workplace, and how negative experiences on the basis of gender identity can be connected to an older feminist literature that problematises the differential and unequal treatment of men and women in places of work (for example, Heilman, 1995). Alex was also able to provide a view of medical practitioner language and behaviour in a context without a patient present:

'We had on one placement I was on ... there was someone who, certainly on records was a man, and who was presenting male, but who had somewhat effeminate mannerisms and a little bit of a high-pitched feminine tone of voice and pattern of speech. Which – so what? And as soon as they [the patient] were gone out the room [nursing colleagues said] – "Do you think that's a woman? I bet that's a woman! I bet it's a woman that's just like – being a man, or it's a tranny!" And I was like "No, if it was someone who was transitioned and was on hormones as you're suggesting then their voice would be lower, surely?" I was trying to like, logic it, because telling your boss that they're a bigot doesn't work. And they were like "Oh maybe they forgot to take their medication this morning." I was like, you can't change someone's voice box in a day by missing your medication!' (Alex, 20, interview)

While power dynamics position patients as being more vulnerable, trans/non-binary staff can be uniquely disenfranchised by cissexist assumptions and gendered (or transphobic) practices from colleagues. In addition, even if successfully performing a professional persona and negotiating a positive interaction with a trans/non-binary service user, cultural practices that allow for the normalisation of slurs (such as 'tranny') and voyeuristic, overt speculation regarding patients' genders are deeply problematic. Such delegitimising practices must be challenged, and their cultural normalisation dismantled, in order for NHS practice to be able to be responsive and sincerely trans/non-binary-sensitive.

The most consistent view among participants was a sense that primary care practitioners were unlikely to understand or be confident over what 'transgender' means, and even less likely to be specifically aware of the existence of non-binary gender identities. Even in the context of studying to become a health professional, Alex said that the general attitude among healthcare staff is:

'As a whole, the attitude is that it's [non-binary identification] not something that's particularly real, it's not something that's particularly important as well. You know, "we don't need to worry about that". People that are trying to maintain their non-binary identity, I feel, are viewed as often sort of causing trouble, trying to get attention, that it's not an okay thing for them to do. Even with doctors who are really understanding, one once said to me "Don't you think you're letting your identity define you a bit?" It's like well, yeah ... it's my identity! But obviously a cis person wouldn't get that. Because they wouldn't have to constantly defend their identity. But the medical establishment seeing it as we are wrong to be trying to defend them all the time – that we're overreacting.' (Alex, 20, interview)

Alex emphasises the differential attitudes of healthcare practitioners to the gender identifications of trans patients, compared to cis patients. While gender when cis is unquestioned, the act of working to claim a gender different from that assigned at birth serves to emphasise gender. From a cisnormative position where no emphasis on gender is needed, this correspondingly may seem to be an 'overemphasis', and would explain the physician's failure to appreciate why Alex raised the topic of gender in order to be accurately recognised and respected.

While binary-oriented trans narratives have an established medical aetiology (through the constructed sexological discourse of transsexualism), non-binary articulations do not, despite current guidelines being worded in such a way that non-binary inclusivity is at least technically possible. Jess has experience of training medical practitioners through activist work, and so, while having not attended personal medical appointments, stated:

> 'I think that probably ninety-nine per cent of clinicians, of doctors, of nurses, whatever, don't know what a non-binary person is, so is therefore very much more likely to get things wrong, to make mistakes, to force somebody into a binary gender and generally behave in a way that is not conducive to the patient's welfare, but is also pretty shitty in other ways. Of the people who know about non-binary, then a lot of people think it might be a phase.' (Jess, 26, interview)

Jess's view that many of the practitioners who are aware of non-binary identities view them as a 'phase' connects with discussion in Chapter 4 – how transgression of binaries can position one as 'unstable', which undermines the status of one's gender as real or meaningful. The medical framework for considering gender essentialises the property of 'being static' for gender, which troubles equal status for those with fluid experiences of gender. Those people whose experiences of (trans)gender fit with the paradigm legitimised by the medical gaze are correspondingly more likely to be afforded belief in their stability and realness. Transgender support networks are well recognised in not only providing emotional support, solidarity and advice, but also highlighting negative medical experiences (particularly in relation to transition-oriented care) so that others may navigate clinics with as little issue as possible, or so as to avoid practitioners who gain a negative reputation (Hines, 2007b; Kosenko et al., 2013).

Beyond the gender identity clinic: experiences of primary and secondary healthcare

Some participants recorded particular experiences of accessing primary healthcare during the diary-keeping period. I will begin by considering examples of primary care that involve what I term 'gendered medicine' – those procedures or experiences which are explicitly gendered in and of themselves through the gendering of bodies and their parts, such as the examination of genitals or breasts. Such healthcare, in this context, is not specifically connected to medical transition. This will be followed by discussion of clinical experiences which are not so explicitly connected to gender – even though perceptions of gender or transgender status still influence the doctor-patient interaction.

Jamie discussed undergoing a cervical smear test in a medical practice that wasn't trans-sensitive, and showed how potentially harmful the gendering of medical processes can be. In their diary, Jamie said "it took a lot of strength to ring a friend when I got home instead of just taking a knife to my wrists" following from this experience with their primary care practice.

Jamie gave a thorough account of their medical experience, which began with their interaction with a member of reception staff. After being addressed by their previous name (a destabilising and unpleasant experience, and triggering of dysphoria) they produced their deed poll to attempt the record change – for the fourth time. Previous attempts by Jamie to formally have their name changed on medical records were not acted on, despite possession of a deed poll, and allowing the practice several months to enact the change. The interaction then involved the receptionist having a telephone call with "patient central", during which (despite the context of a first name change and gendered title change to 'Mr') Jamie was referred to as "a lady", "she" and "her". While a more detailed consideration of the role of administrative processes in medical care will be considered later in this chapter, this context is important because of the emotional impact of the interaction on Jamie *before* entering the space of the examination room, and the gendered negotiations with the nurse performing the cervical smear.

Jamie made a point of telling the nurse in the examination room that they are transgender. However, the nurse gave no clear indication of having registered or understood the relevance of this for the interaction. Instead she simply continued by replying "Okay. Have you ever used sex toys? It [the speculum used during screenings] is no bigger than a dildo..." This gave Jamie considerable anxiety, uncertain whether the nurse "thinks I was assigned male at birth and have had lower surgery and am worried about my neovagina being hurt or something". While the nurse did express sympathy in response to perceiving anxiety, Jamie characterised her response as very general in nature and did not suggest awareness that Jamie's specific (dysphoric) anxiety was informed by being trans, being misgendered, and the lack of practitioner awareness.

Further, the symbolic use of sex toys to make a point about the speculum is noteworthy. In terms of making the point about size, the nurse could have easily shown the speculum, making the intimate question unnecessary.[4] While inappropriate conduct has been explored in women's healthcare (Moore et al., 2000), the specific context of trans/non-binary carries different requirements for sensitive practice, which has lacked specific discussion within existing literature. Arguably, the speculum–dildo comparison also connects sex toys and trans status through a discourse of sexual deviance. Most problematically is how Jamie recounted the exchange during physical examination:

> Nurse: So how do you cope with your period?
>
> Me (thinking, WHAT THE FUCK?! Why do you think this is a) appropriate or b) at all likely to calm me down?! Are you seriously trying to dispel my anxiety by bringing up the precise dysphoria I'm currently desperately trying to dispel?!?!?!): Badly. (Jamie, 24, diary, emphasis original)

This illustrates unambiguously how practitioners' inappropriate interactions can cause extreme discomfort, stemming from lack of awareness regarding trans/non-binary needs. The phrasing of the question, and the fact that the nurse did not ask for any more information following Jamie's response of "badly" suggests that this question was not asked out of medical necessity. The inaccurate collapse of 'people with cervixes' to the social category of 'woman' results in a blanket-style approach to particular healthcare interactions that have the potential to be delegitimising and upsetting.

Mark's discussion of his (gendered, but not GIC-related) secondary care experiences with a gynaecologist provides another perspective:

'On paper, I'm very scary apparently, I'm told. [According to] the gynaecologist that was checking me out ... I'm having trouble with my digestive system actually, but when it first came up it was assumed to be an ovary. So that meant a trip to the gynaecologist. And he apparently, somebody really hadn't felt very comfortable dealing with me ... and I thought "what's wrong with me?" but I think when I get in there and they realise that I'm first of all quite personable, I'm not kind of going in grunting. I don't have the testosterone sweats or anything like that! And also, that I'm happy within the contexts of what they're doing to be open about being transgender. I had another ultrasound recently; they're trying to tick off what's not wrong with me at the moment, anyway. But of course, the lady doing the ultrasound wanted to know what the background was, had I been for one recently, yes, I went for one before Christmas, but that was specifically just to check my ovaries. Because I'm transgender, and that was fine. That was the only conversation that went on about it. But I think if they realised that I go in and I don't have two heads, that hopefully there's a weird sort of educational process going on! That just because someone called Mark is coming in to have their ovaries looked at doesn't mean I'm going to be a monster.' (Mark, 43, interview)

Mark is keen to emphasise that through being personable, he is able to dispel much of the anxiety that practitioners expressed in relation to him. It is important to recognise the significance of the gynaecologist telling Mark, his patient, that he found him to be 'very scary on paper', and the additional emotional labour necessary from Mark to manage his healthcare interactions. Through Mark's possession and embodiment of a trans history, this is enough in and of itself to cause fear in the clinician. One interpretation of this fear is discomfort with Mark, on the basis that 'trans status is scary'. This has been explored through feelings of transgender rage at being positioned as an artificial creation, and monstrously different (Stryker, 1994; Nordmarken, 2014). Alternatively/additionally, the doctor's fear may have been over worrying about potentially failing to provide adequate care – the fear of failing as a physician (McLeod, 2003).

These two examples from Mark and Jamie illustrate significant narrative differences, in that Mark did not express being upset by how his treatment was conducted or the nature of the practitioner's communication, while Jamie did. This may be related to *trans time* from Chapter 4, in that Jamie was in the early stages of negotiating their identity while Mark articulated considerably more experience and security. Further, Mark's doctor did explicitly recognise him as trans, and engaged in a recognisable act of rapport building (however problematic). The response of Jamie's nurse to Jamie's act of coming out in the clinical space was symbolic erasure (Namaste, 2000), through failing to respond in a way that demonstrated trans status was intelligible, and the subsequent upsetting questions.

As Mark had his name already registered and used consistently at the doctor's (and with his name being read unambiguously as male), this was an unmissable marker for medical staff. The difference also meant that Mark did not share Jamie's experience of trying to have the correct name and title arranged (yet again) before the appointment in question, which in Jamie's case, primed vulnerability. Further, due to having already accessed gender-affirming medical services, Mark was read socially as male more consistently than Jamie – making it considerably easier for Mark to avoid being assumed to be female, even within the setting of a gynaecological examination. Mark explained that earlier in his transition, he was more easily upset and destabilised by the behaviours of clinicians:

'A couple of times I have made complaints to practice managers, but that was generally in the very early days. And the trouble is of course, back when ... you have so little to hang on to. You have no testosterone, no surgery, you are basically told to get out there and be a man.' (Mark, 43, interview)

This adds to the temporally and materially dependent discourse of 'not being trans enough' as discussed in Chapter 3. There is potential insecurity in not feeling (or being viewed as) trans enough, when an individual has not yet accessed (or does not intend to access) transition-related treatment. Further, individuals may feel they lacked the catalysis of embodied change, which would not only stimulate confidence in one's trans modality, but also allow for less problematic negotiation of (gendered) services. Unless a trans person who is accessing gendered medicine exhibits unambiguous social markers of cross-gender identification or embodiment, their identity, and correspondingly their particular socio-medical needs may be rendered invisible if nuanced trans-sensitive policy and staff training are not in place.

In terms of misgendering, many participants expressed how being read as 'the binary gender converse to their assignment' is considerably preferable. Avoiding being positioned as the gender that one was 'assigned' without medical 'intervention' can be difficult for some and impossible for others. Thus, presenting oneself in accordance with one's assigned gender can be a survival mechanism for navigating the world with fewer practical difficulties. In such cases, the individual's gendered appearance is taken at face value, due to medicine operating within cisnormative society whereby appearance functions as 'cultural genitals' (Kessler and McKenna, 1978). Which of these two undesirable options is taken may depend on the severity of dysphoria – which can vary not only between different people, but with time (and triggers) for individuals.

Only when the medical record of 'M' or 'F', and gendered appearance are 'misaligned enough' does an individual have a chance of being regularly recognised as trans within medical contexts. Lack of non-binary-specific markers means this will near-universally be in binary terms, although it is also possible that staff may instead presume the gender marker on records to be a 'mistake'. The potential confusion that trans embodiment can cause is also supported by Frankie's account of receiving an ultrasound, after experiencing abdominal pain since starting HRT:

> The clinician was nice enough, just kinda did his thing and then I left. I got the impression he might have been slightly flustered about how to treat me, looking 'male' but with 'female' details – think there were a couple of questions where he really thought about the wording before asking, which was cool. (Frankie, 25, diary)

The symbolic disjuncture between appearance and records (as with Mark) acted as a social cue which the doctor was able to recognise, and modify his interaction accordingly. Frankie's account also illustrates how recognising the act of the doctor thinking about how to word his questions may help trans/non-binary people feel more at ease, as recognising such an action is evidence of concern for the patient in terms of their trans/non-binary status. It provides evidence of a practitioner with some awareness of gender sensitivity and, importantly, an active desire to be respectful and create an affirming environment.

To compare this interaction with Jamie's smear test, Jamie may have avoided some elements of distress had their earlier attempts to change their records been successful, but the interaction with the nurse was partly due to her assumption that Jamie was female. However, her inappropriate question about how Jamie 'copes with [their] periods', asked in the context of *knowing* Jamie's trans status, was not rooted in medical necessity (but rather, curiosity), and did not recognise the potential sensitivity of the situation as Frankie's clinician did. This illustrates how trans/non-binary clinical experience may have a significantly unpredictable element to it, dependent on the personality and style of a given practitioner. While this may also be true from a practitioner perspective (in that trans/non-binary service users are very heterogeneous and therefore not predictable), there is a great sense of concordance from trans communities regarding modes of practice that are viewed as sensitive, collaborative, and preferable (Dewey, 2008, 2013; Ellis et al., 2014, 2015).

In relation to uterine and sexual healthcare experiences, Ash drew an image of their internal reproductive structures in order to clarify 'what they had' (Figure 7).

This image literally illustrates non-binary embodiment, and the results of negotiation both with oneself and with the providers of medical care. The image shows at least two independent medical procedures – testicular implants, and an intrauterine device. In gendered terms, such procedures would typically be assumed as mutually exclusive. Therefore, this highlights both the introspective work done in reaching the decision of wanting a non-binary

Figure 7: Illustration of non-binary vagina with prosthetic testicles and intrauterine device, from Ash's diary

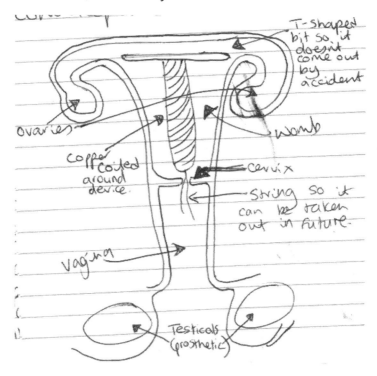

physiology, and the effort required to successfully access this through appeals to both identification (Baril and Trevenen, 2014) and sexual responsibility and autonomy.

In addition to the impact of clinician awareness, sensitivity and demeanour, explanations related to health and diagnoses given by doctors have interplay with gender identity. Within their diary, Ash talked about sometimes feeling that their reproductive system might be "broken, not as good as that of cisgender people". Ash here illustrates internalisation of the stigma of a body that does not fulfil idealised (cis)gendered expectations. The rendering of the physiological in moral terms ('not as good') fuses two of Goffman's (1997: 205) types of stigma: "abominations of the body" and "blemishes of individual character", both of which are relatable to trans embodiment.

Ash's feelings of being lesser or damaged related to their experience of sexual healthcare, as well as their history of receiving HRT. Ash discussed having a contraceptive copper coil fitted and explained how it tends to make menstrual flow heavier, meaning they were bleeding more than they had for years. Contrary to experiencing dysphoria in relation to this (as would be expected of a hegemonic AFAB trans narrative), Ash explained they were happy about this, because it made them feel less 'broken'. The coil served to reduce anxiety Ash had over a perceived increased risk of cancer:

When I went to see an endocrinologist and they put me on female hormones I asked why I have to do 3 weeks on, 1 week off cycle when lots of people (trans women) I know take oestrogen every day of every month. The endocrinologist said if you have a womb it is different. You should take time off oestrogen to let your womb bleed. If your womb does not shed its lining regularly this is bad for you, and you are at greater risk of cancer. So after they said that I have often looked at the tiny red smear in my knickers each month and felt anxious that it's not enough and I will get cancer. (Ash, 33, diary)

The act of menstruating, rather than being a simple cause of dysphoria (as it may or may not have been in Ash's past) reassured Ash that their physiology was 'working', and so it felt to them less likely that they were at risk of uterus-related pathology. Oestrogen-only HRT may increase the risk of womb cancer (Grady et al., 1995), and is therefore only recommended for AFAB people who have had a hysterectomy (NHS, 2016). However, combined HRT of oestrogen and progesterone *reduces* cancer risk (Hill et al., 2000). The Faculty of Sexual & Reproductive Healthcare (FSRH) of the Royal College of Obstetricians & Gynaecologists has advised that there is no health benefit from taking a seven-day break from the combined contraceptive pill (BBC News, 2019). Therefore, as Ash's endocrinologist would have known they had a womb (and was thus contraindicated for oestrogen-only HRT, such that Ash should have received a combination prescription), their claim about the need for time off the pill was factually incorrect. The anxiety this produced for Ash creates a complex intersection with gender identity.

Gender could be unnecessarily brought to bear even in very mundane medical interactions. Alex illustrated this by explaining in their diary how, when expressing discomfort at a local anaesthetic injection for the removal of an ingrown toenail, the nurse practitioner said "Once women have babies they don't complain anymore." While the nurse's response implied that she was being glib, one could argue that regardless of the patient's gender this response may be interpreted as dismissive (and essentially a way of saying 'stop complaining'). When Alex responded by saying they were never going to have children, the nurse responded with "the usual patronising line about how I'm young and I'd change my mind one day". Alex communicated finding this annoying to the nurse. Although the nurse did not verbally respond, Alex reported feeling a sense of "judgement and disapproval". It is important to note that such an interaction may have been equally offensive to many cisgender women, due to the stereotypical assumption of those read as women inevitably being positioned as (future) mothers. However, the way in which such an interaction also can heighten dysphoria and delegitimise an individual's gender identity entirely, means this has particular significance in the context of trans/non-binary interactions. As a student nurse with first-hand experience of how medical professionals are taught and expected to behave in a non-judgemental manner, Alex was particularly critical of this interaction. This instance not only reinforces how gender norms and expectations can be clinically reified, but how they can be brought to the fore even when there is no gendered element to the health concern being addressed.

The following health concern (a sore arm) from Mark was conflated with his gender-related medical treatment and dismissed. Binary-oriented and non-binary trans people who access gender-affirming medical interventions can find unrelated health experiences being consigned to 'side effects' of, for example, HRT:

> I have had a sore arm for around 4 years. It actually
> started before I first took T. I went to see a doctor
> about the pain after a couple of years (you can't accuse
> me of over-extending the NHS!) and was told that the
> muscles in my arm were growing, due to the T, and
> that these were essentially 'growing pains'. "But why
> just in one arm?" I queried. The reply was that as I
> am right handed, I was using the 'new' muscles more
> frequently, so wasn't experiencing pain. In my poor,
> slovenly left arm, I had pain due to my body not being
> used to the muscle growth. At that point I gave up.
> (Mark, 43, diary)

Mark specifies that his arm pain began before he ever took testosterone,
yet the explanation he received relied on his prescription as causation.
Further, the explanation is clearly unsatisfactory for Mark, yet he
chose to 'give up', due to the sense that attempting to challenge the
doctor's position further would be too demanding, and likely produce
no results. There are parallels here with how other stigmatised patients
receive inappropriate medical scrutiny and blame, such as when a
patient is overweight (Foster et al., 2003).

Mark can be understood to be negotiating his relationship with
his doctors so as to fulfil the role of the 'good patient' (Lorber,
1975), reducing the risk of conflict. This was also seen in how
Mark navigated his interactions with the gynaecologist, working to
perform a particularly amenable persona in order to counteract and
diffuse any apprehensions a physician may have over trans patients
being 'difficult'. This could be both in terms of how to treat, and
in terms of patient behaviour as challenging or disrupting the
doctor's presumed superiority in the context of the clinic. Mark
also previously mentioned his hope that "there's a weird sort of
educational process going on", illustrating how by performing the
role of an agreeable patient he hopes to further normalise trans
people to his clinicians.

Another very different account of gender transition intersecting with
additional health concerns was described by Ash:

> A couple of years ago I kept pointing out to my doctor
> that I had the symptoms of severe malnutrition and the
> doctor wasn't helpful at all – just kept saying "eat xyz",
> which I was already eating. I was really ill. The only
> thing that made it stop was the GP being confused by my

gender, and saying he wasn't willing to prescribe HRT until I'd seen an endocrinologist and they had said it was appropriate ... I am so lucky that being transgender got me diagnosed and treated appropriately in this indirect way. I am pissed off that they didn't take me seriously earlier and I had to feel ill for a couple of years for no good reason ... During this time I actually went into hospital and had a blood transfusion because I had so few red blood cells (anaemia) on two separate occasions. They were saying "you must've been bleeding heavily, how did this happen?" and they didn't believe me when I said I hadn't. (Ash, 33, diary)

Ash explains how they felt lucky that their gender transition meant that they were treated appropriately for the nutrient deficiencies they had; however, it is problematic that this wasn't followed up in its own right. This example doesn't suggest it is appropriate practice for secondary care referrals (rather than a simple blood test) to be necessarily required prior to HRT prescription. Ash needed to be seen by an endocrinologist, but not because of wishing to start HRT. The assumptions within medicine that bodies which are gendered a particular way perform similarly (in this case, that people with wombs must bleed) meant that Ash felt medical staff distrusted them, rather than entertaining the possibility of another explanation. The importance of practitioners trusting patients has been explored (Peter and Watt-Watson, 2002; Rogers, 2002), which is particularly valuable in cases with relatively frequent, ongoing contact such as with cases of chronic illness (Thorne et al., 2000).

Disability, chronic illness and being non-binary

The last example with Ash highlights how a patient's condition(s) – in that case, a history of mental health diagnoses – can potentially have an impact on interactions with medical practitioners. Intersections between experiences of disability and chronic illness were raised by multiple participants, and how this affected their negotiations of non-binary gender identity. Further, the impact of medical interactions was multifaceted. Mark explained in his diary how he experiences multiple chronic conditions:

Of my medical files ...
Bipolar (Type 2 – I take lithium)

Hypothyroidism (caused by lithium. Crap)
OCD (The diagnosed sort, not the trendy one)
Gout (bloody painful)
IBS (maybe – the doctor isn't sure)
GENDER DYSPHORIA (well, duh) (Mark, 43, diary,
emphasis original)

Mark wrote how this meant he had a lot of experience with doctors, as well as being "well known" at his local surgery. This was to such an extent that "the pharmacist just hands over my drugs without asking my name". Mark further contextualises how his mother was a nurse, so he is "not scared" of medics. Contrary to this, Ricky's chronic health problems alienated (rather than acclimatised) them from doctors. Ricky detailed how they were diagnosed with ME[5] in 1998, and how their related experiences soured them towards the medical profession. Their determination to access hormones despite this aversion (and the symptomatic fatigue of their condition) helped Ricky realise to themselves how serious they were, and thus how significant gendered medical interventions were for them. They went on to explain how:

> 'We're really lucky where we are, because we live in this tiny little old mining village. And it's got a tiny little GP practice which they've never managed to find a GP to take it over, so it's been locums for years. We've got a guy there now who's been the locum there for a really long time. But he's one of those doctors that you just go in, you tell him what you want and he gives it to you. He's not really that interested, he's just got his feet up, he's very laid back, and you just go in and go "I'm trans, refer me to the gender clinic," and he goes "Okay," and he writes a letter, and you tell him what to write – I can live with that level of interaction. If I actually needed a GP that was going to help me and talk stuff through with me and investigate something or put their own thoughts into what was going on for me, I think I'd be really stuffed. But as long as I know what I need, then I can get it.' (Ricky, 43, interview)

Ricky's earlier medical interactions firmly shaped how they wished to interact with medical practitioners – both in relation to chronic illness, and gender identity. They recognise how their GP's apparent apathy can be problematised, though Ricky self-describes as 'lucky' – because of the fit between their doctor's approach and their individual needs and preferences. Ricky's experiences of being chronically ill prepared them for assuming the role of the expert patient (Taylor and Bury, 2007), so as to claim power in accessing what they felt they needed:

'There's no point going to them and saying "I'm feeling this, can you help me," I have to go "I need this from you." I think in some ways that's also a process of empowerment, really, and has certainly helped with being trans. I didn't go along to the doctor and go "You know I think I might be" or "I think this is going on", I just went and said "You need to refer me to the gender clinic please," and I think that's quite empowering from that point of view. With my ME I had to take it into my own hands, I realised the medical profession just didn't have answers for me.' (Ricky, 43, interview)

The way Ricky represented themselves through their language as confident and certain of their needs discursively aligns with stability and validity – and thus greater chance of validation by the medical gaze. Diagnosis with gender dysphoria is dependent on trans individuals self-reporting, such that expressing lack of confidence in the claim (or being read as such, for whatever reason) may produce clinical doubt in the service-user, in primary care or GIC contexts.

Jess explained how her experience of being disabled shapes how she is symbolically read, and thus how she is interacted with. Initially, Jess contextualised how her impairment affects her speech and gait, such that she went through both speech therapy and physiotherapy during childhood. Jess articulates that these aspects of her expression that are positioned as "markers of [her] queerness" – their 'mincing walk' and 'gay voice' – are for her, markers of disability:

'I feel like my identity as a disabled person is quite often subsumed into my queerness, and kind of consumed by it. It means that a lot of the time I'm not seen as disabled at all, which can be quite difficult when I need to access disability-specific things, or talk about disabled people. People see it as being about my queerness. And that's probably because it makes me look physically queer. Which obviously puts me in danger, and allows me easier access to queer spaces ... I think that partially it's the disability, those disability markers are being read as femininity, this means that I'm kind of often misgendered as being a femme when what they mean is you're a femme boy, rather than a kind of butch woman. I've also noticed that as another interesting intersection between disability and transness is that I get a significantly less amount of harassment when I'm walking with my walking stick than when I'm not. So, I often feel like sometimes even if I don't need it, I might take my walking stick out. Because it feels a bit like a foil, people see the stick and don't look at you. You've already been classified as a disabled person rather than as a trans person or a gender freak or whatever. It's like people can only see you as one thing. It means that in general I get an easier time of it. So especially if I'm going on long journeys on public transport, I'll take my stick, even if I don't need it, because public transport seems to be where most of my misgendering and harassment and sexual assaults and violence happens against me but seems to happen less often if I'm walking with my stick.' (Jess, 26, interview)

Jess felt that her walk and speech contributed to her being coded by others as 'queer' more so than 'disabled', compounded by social actors erroneously assuming she is 'male' via appearance (Sandahl, 2003; Whitney, 2006). That is, gendered assumptions potentially alter the symbolic ascription of meaning to embodied traits, which may simultaneously create risk, and signal belonging. By encouraging a disability reading through her use of the stick, Jess can feel protected against transphobic abuse.

Rachel included material in their diary raising intersections with their experiences as a disabled person (Figures 8, 9, 10).

Jess may mitigate experiences of harassment through socially positioning herself in a manner which results in her gendered presentation being explained away, rather than punished, which resonates with Rachel's sense that social actors symbolically ascribe disability as the explanation for 'gender-inappropriate' presentation. That disabled people are often socially positioned as either not experiencing or not understanding sexual desire is an ableist trope that is well recognised (Di Giulio, 2003). The text overlay in Rachel's image (Figure 8) highlights potential insecurity in relation to genderqueer identification. As Rachel did not highlight experiencing any cognitive impairment, this question is likely rhetorical, as those who are physically disabled often experience being patronised (Stevens, 2014), and treated as if mentally impaired and unable to make 'appropriate' choices by themselves. There is an important intersectional consideration in Rachel's account, as while disabled people may struggle to find clothes that are comfortable, accessible and stylish, a trans identity adds additional constraints to clothing choice. For example, a gendered clothing cut may cause pain due to tightness,

Figure 8: Image of disabled individuals in wheelchairs, from Rachel's diary

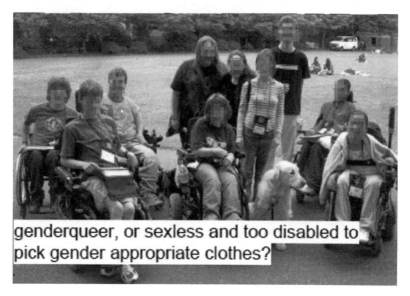

or gendered clothing may differ in the difficulty to put on and take off relative to the individual's body.

Rachel's experiences of chronic illness and their experiences of gender cannot be disentangled, in terms of medical treatment as well as social interactions. The opiates which Rachel was taking during the diary-keeping period served to relieve their gender dysphoria, though were not prescribed in relation to this. Rachel explained how they did not wish to discuss gender with their doctors because they feared it may disrupt their other carefully managed and highly necessary healthcare interventions. This was also Bobby's approach to navigating their chronic (mental) healthcare:

> Naturally I have not told [the mental health team] any gender stuff ... they would almost certainly latch onto any hint of gender identity and DECIDE that everything I'm going through, all of the mental health issues, all of it is entirely based in gender... They will think of my gender identity as either the cause or result or both of this crisis. (Bobby, 23, diary, emphasis original)

Illness or disability may synergise with perceptions of healthcare providers to create additional healthcare barriers. Access to mental health care can be limited when stigmatisation of mental health

Figure 9: Image of pills, from Rachel's diary

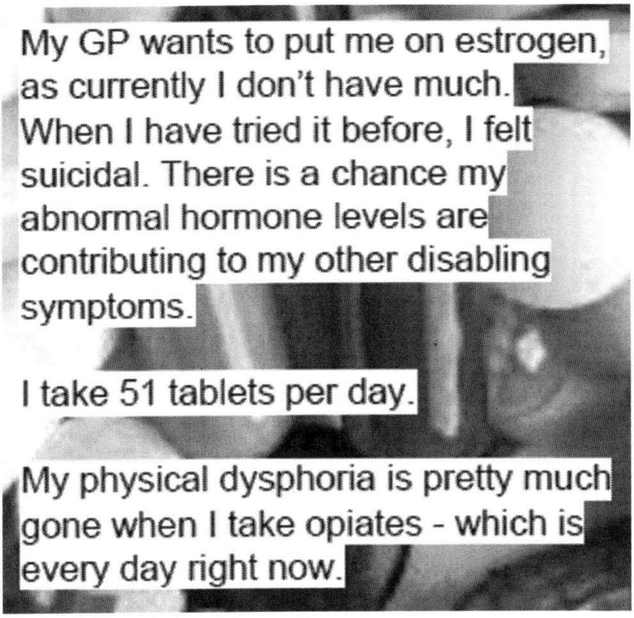

My GP wants to put me on estrogen, as currently I don't have much. When I have tried it before, I felt suicidal. There is a chance my abnormal hormone levels are contributing to my other disabling symptoms.

I take 51 tablets per day.

My physical dysphoria is pretty much gone when I take opiates - which is every day right now.

conditions is feared or expected, which is likely to be exacerbated by intersectional fear/expectation of trans stigma. Rachel said that "If I can put up with them seeing me as female and using those pronouns and stuff it seems like a better option," because of the risks, and the associated labour (in explaining their feelings to service providers for potentially no gain). Rachel's healthcare management can also be linked back to how experiences of non-binary gender is temporally dependent – as Rachel's experience of dysphoria is significantly different depending on the medication they are or are not taking at a given time.

Figure 10 illustrates how chronic illness and disability can constrain not only access to discussing gender or medical transition with doctors, but also gender presentation, and therefore social interactions. Relating back to Figure 2, where Rachel stated 'I feel like a man trapped inside a woman's body. Except the body is comfy and pretty and safe' shows that there are multiple aspects to Rachel's experiences of embodiment that coexist in tension with each other. These tensions do not undermine the validity of Rachel's identity, but serve to illustrate how different facets can hold greater or lesser significance in a manner dependent on context and time. Rachel iterates that changing the way they dress to better match their identity actually makes them feel *worse*,

Figure 10: Image of breasts in bra, from Rachel's diary

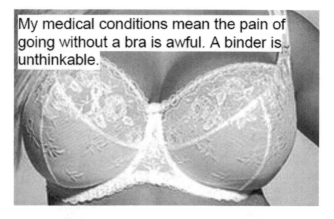

My medical conditions mean the pain of going without a bra is awful. A binder is unthinkable.

as the disjunction between their physicality and gendered presentation serves to emphasise that they are 'trapped inside a woman's body'. This serves to disrupt hegemonic narratives of transgender embodiment, which can lack space for experiences from, for example, AFAB people who do not bind their breasts, presenting in a manner that is culturally consistent with feminine expectation. Such traits, as well as experience of chronic illness (ME, as with Ricky), were shared by Charlie.

Chronic health conditions and disability influence the relationships individuals have with the medical profession. Treatments themselves may also significantly affect the experiences of gender dysphoria and/ or gender identity, which feed into negotiations of the social world. The relationship between chronic health conditions and (not) being referred to a GIC could manifest in different ways, as it did for Ricky and Rachel. The important administrative process of referral by a GP together with the impact of other clerical interactions will now be considered.

Medical administration: being referred, being frustrated

In primary care, experiences with non-medical staff and with administrative systems themselves can pose specific difficulties for non-binary people. Jamie's difficulty procuring a name and title change highlighted the potential difficulties and distress that can be encountered when negotiating administrative processes within one's medical practice. Following a six-month wait, Jamie gave the practice an ultimatum, threatening to report them to the Patient Advice and Liaison Service (PALS – which supports formal complaint proceedings within the NHS):

They rang me on the last day of my ultimatum to say 'I don't know if you know, but it's very complicated what we have to do, we have to get a new NHS number' I know! I gave you the guidance of what to do! Don't tell me what you have to do as if I don't understand how complicated it was. (Jamie, 24, diary)

The nature of this interaction follows a parallel narrative to that of the 'expert patient' (Taylor and Bury, 2007), which subverts power dynamics through challenging and resisting the supposed expertise of the professional – typically the clinician, but here the administrator. This expands the role and knowledge of the expert patient beyond healthcare decision making, such that an individual becomes a 'manager patient'. I use this term to refer to contexts where, rather than (only) demonstrating significant familiarity with medical literature and expert status in relation to trans healthcare, the patient performs managerial labour in guiding and instructing medical staff in administrative processes. Thus, 'expert status' can extend beyond the doctor-patient interaction, due to the significance of gender in record keeping that does not intersect with other examples of expert patients. However, the patient still lacks the power to enforce their knowledge of institutional policy, and remains dependent on staff following their instruction – which, as Jamie's circumstance demonstrates, cannot be depended on.

This altercation highlights the inadequacy of the current system in allowing for record changes. This is not only due to the complexity of the task itself, but the failure by administration to recognise that the delay in making the change may produce significant distress. Leon also experienced problems, specifically stating in their diary that "The practice won't seem to let me go by my preferred name". This could suggest a lack of transparency in the name change protocol making it difficult for Leon to access, or inconsistency between the policies of different clinics. It also raises the question of clinic policy on recording preferred names (for waiting room announcements and interactions), and whether administrative systems are built to be able to accommodate this universally. The potential impact of dysphoria and stress through administrative delays and the excessive patient labour this can demand is emphasised through Jamie's statement that "It's been really stressful and horrible, because it definitely puts me off going to the doctor. It nearly put me off going for a mole which has now been diagnosed as possibly melanoma."

Conversely, Mark indicated he was impressed with the clinic's sensitivity of communication (from the position of having had his gender marker and name successfully changed on his medical records):

> The letter was addressed to Mr. [surname], and used impeccable language, which I suspect took someone some time to formulate, given that I am a Mr. with a uterus and ovaries. (Mark, 43, diary)

Mark praises the nameless staff member who wrote the letter for respecting his title and pronouns in a context of writing about his uterus and ovaries, stressing the awareness of how the social possibility of 'a Mr with a uterus and ovaries' is rarely recognised. Mark's satisfaction may also potentially be influenced by the extensive misgendering that practically all trans people experience. Contexts such as this, where the respect, and, by proxy, social legitimacy of gender identity are threatened (in this case through the explicit juxtaposition with physiology) may result in relief when misgendering doesn't happen. In a sense, Mark may be grateful for a level of nuance rarely found outside transgender communities, which contrasts with the frustration that other participants articulate when expecting and experiencing administrative misgendering. This example also demonstrates how a non-binary identity is not a reliable predictor of title (or pronoun) usage, with Mark using 'he' and 'Mr', rather than 'they', and 'Mx'.

The fact that Mark's administrative markers of name, pronouns and title are all socially coded as 'male' likely assist in consistent and aware administration, in comparison to using the title 'Mx' or singular they as a pronoun. Mark also further evidences performing the role of a 'good patient' in an administrative as well as clinical setting, through deliberately articulating a presentation that is more feminine or camp than he generally would. This affectation serves not only to position him as non-threatening to reception staff 'Trying Very Hard to be nonchalant' (note the deliberate capitalisation for emphasis from the diary entry), but also to assist in the negotiation of his own comfort levels within the setting of gendered medicine. In performing himself as a feminine male, Mark recodes himself twice over to ease the symbolic dissonance staff may experience between his identity and embodiment.

Despite being broadly comfortable with being socially read and positioned as male in navigating day-to-day life, Mark explicitly states feeling uncomfortable as male in the gynaecologist's office, alluding potentially to how the space is socially constructed as 'for women'. While an explanation in terms of dysphoria is also possible, it is problematic to assume this as a/the source of Mark's discomfort, and would risk further reinforcing the clinically constructed, hegemonic, binarised narrative of gender dysphoria.

Frankie used their diary to share their thoughts and feelings concerning administration, particularly through engagement with feedback forms. Frankie shared photographs they had taken of forms they had completed after attending particular secondary and tertiary care appointments.

As Figure 11 shows, Frankie rated their overall satisfaction with their experience of receiving an ultrasound 'excellent', although they did also point out in the additional comments section how the binary tick boxes for gender did not provide them with an acceptable option for their identity at that time. The second image (Figure 12) was taken of a feedback form following an appointment with a GIC. While Frankie's views on such care will be further explored in the next chapter, this feedback form illustrates how the only aspect of Frankie's experience that was particularly problematic was that of administrative staff. While Frankie felt involved in their treatment and broadly confident in their clinician(s), there remained aspects of respectfulness and ability to listen that could be improved on, despite offering overall positive feedback.

Secondary and tertiary care contexts produce forms for the collection of healthcare-related information that is more specific than primary clinical needs. However, Jamie's discussion of one such form highlighted significant problems with its construction and resultant impact, as discussed in Chapter 3. The length of the form meant a larger burden was placed on patients who were required to complete it, and the ambiguous or uncertain purpose of some questions inspired anxiety. Jamie highlights how the psychopathological construction of gender dysphoria has led to clinical assumptions that feelings about

Figure 11: Scan of secondary care clinical feedback form, from Frankie's diary

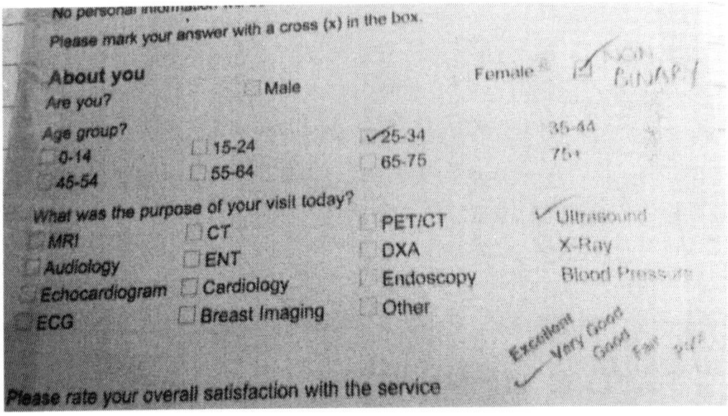
Please mark your answer with a cross (x) in the box.

About you

Are you? Male Female NON BINARY

Age group?
0-14 15-24 25-34 35-44
45-54 55-64 65-75 75+

What was the purpose of your visit today?
MRI CT PET/CT Ultrasound
Audiology ENT DXA X-Ray
Echocardiogram Cardiology Endoscopy Blood Pressure
ECG Breast Imaging Other

Excellent Very Good Good Fair Poor

Please rate your overall satisfaction with the service

Figure 12: Scan of GIC feedback form, from Frankie's diary

1. The administrative staff were pleasant and respectful.	Strongly Agree	Agree	Neither Agree Nor Disagree	Disagree (circled)	Strongly Disagree
2. The clinician was pleasant and respectful.	Strongly Agree	Agree (circled)	Neither Agree Nor Disagree	Disagree	Strongly Disagree
3. I feel listened to.	Strongly Agree	Agree (circled)	Neither Agree Nor Disagree	Disagree	Strongly Disagree
4. I feel involved in my treatment.	Strongly Agree (circled)	Agree	Neither Agree Nor Disagree	Disagree	Strongly Disagree
5. I have confidence in the abilities of the clinician.	Strongly Agree (circled)	Agree	Neither Agree Nor Disagree	Disagree	Strongly Disagree
6. I am likely to recommend this service/team to friends or family if they need similar care or treatment.	Strongly Agree (circled)	Agree	Neither Agree Nor Disagree	Disagree	Strongly Disagree
7. The information was provided in a way that was understandable.	Strongly Agree (circled)	Agree	Neither Agree Nor Disagree	Disagree	Strongly Disagree
8. Any questions I had were answered.	Strongly Agree (circled)	Agree	Neither Agree Nor Disagree	Disagree	Strongly Disagree

parts of the body can be articulated in simple positive or negative terms, that can be essentialised to 33 specific body parts.[6] Jamie demonstrated in their diary how flaws in the form's design render it vulnerable to deconstruction and ambiguous interpretation.

Jamie's discussion within their diary showed they were scrutinising the questions to assess the purpose for which they were being asked, but was anxious due to lack of transparency from the GIC concerning how such information might be used by medical practitioners. For example, on reading questions asking whether the individual felt their buttocks were too big, Jamie interpreted this as potentially screening for the presence of an eating disorder, which could then jeopardise being seen as 'really trans'. This provides an example of a phenomenon already observed within binary-oriented trans navigations of GICs – significant anxiety concerning how clinicians make their assessments, and a desire to fulfil expectations (by performing the role of 'good patient') as closely as possible, so as to successfully access desired outcomes.

For non-binary people this is particularly difficult, as non-binary identification in itself can be constituted by some practitioners as less certain, more complicated, and lacking historical precedence.

The presentation within the form inspired feelings from Jamie in the diary that 'they seem like terrifying unknowns designed to trip you up, to trick you into revealing that you're not trans at all'. This resonates with how Jess described her sense of GIC care provision processes:

> 'It is incredibly pathologising and essentially assumes that the person being referred to them is a cis person who is having some sort of delusions. The kind of process isn't a process of affirming people's genders but is a process of trying to 'catch out' the secret cis people who are deluded enough to go through this process. And in that way obviously the trans healthcare system is actually entirely built around cis people, and 'saving' cis people from becoming trans. Which is one of the reasons why it's particularly bad for non-binary people, because people have a particularly binary-focused way of understanding what trans is, and so if you show any deviation from a binary transition pathway or a binary life then you're likely to be seen as a deluded cis person.' (Jess, 26, interview)

That Jamie recounted how their trans community group engaged in a particular discussion of the GIC's form illustrates how members of gender-diverse communities can function to assist each other in navigating healthcare. This can influence which clinics trans people choose to access, as Finn described:

> 'I've got a [GP] who is more trans friendly/actually knows what to do. So I'm going to ask them to refer me to [particular GIC], because I recently made a trans friend who has had a really good experience there. They were seen in a lot shorter time, one of his clinicians is trans and I was like "Wow that sounds so much better." And I have a friend in [city] who I'd be able to stay with if I needed to.' (Finn, 22, interview)

Thus, Finn's decision to access a particular clinic was directly informed by the experience from a trans friend. The reputations of clinics (and individual clinicians) spread within trans networks so as to influence patterns of access.

The remainder of this chapter relates to experiences and views of the referral process from primary to secondary care. It is not necessary for GPs to make any form of assessment before referring people who make such a request to GICs. Guidelines simply state 'those who need gender identity services for the first time should be referred by the GP' (Wylie et al., 2014: 172). However, there was a sense among participants that getting referred could be an unnecessarily arduous process. Jamie stated that their GP felt that "it was important [for him to ask questions], 'I'm only going to refer you if you tell me that you've felt like this for years and years' so I lied". In this context, 'it' was the sense that there was a perceived need by the GP to ask questions – by the GP's understanding, the GP's role was that of gatekeeper to specialist services. When considering referral to secondary or tertiary medical services more generally, this is rooted in a UK-specific historical context of demand management (Loudon, 2008). The ethics regarding gatekeeping practices have been considered, with the potential for under-referral to save medical resources, or over-referral in private 'for-profit' care being particularly problematised (Pellegrino, 1986). The complete absence of inherent pathology in the specific case of trans identification fundamentally differentiates gender identity-related medical interventions from other healthcare referrals. Increasing recognition of this through education and trans service-user demands is bringing the role of the GP into debate (Singh and Burnes, 2010). There was a sense that when GPs are asked to provide referrals, they would be unfamiliar with the gender dysphoria pathway:

> 'They generally don't have any idea about trans stuff. You know, they're reluctant to do stuff like referring you to GICs, to monitor you once they get you back, to even treat you for other medical stuff because they get side-tracked by trans stuff.' (Rachel, 28, interview)

> 'So then I went to the GP here, who was utterly clueless about ... she said outright "I've never had a trans patient," in some convoluted way, like "I have never had a transgender"!' (Leon, 34, interview)

Leon's implicit frustration here is not just with the "utterly clueless" GP, but with the circumstances that mean managing the relationship with their GP somewhat depends on their ability to reassure the GP that 'that's okay!'. I argue that being personable when faced with professional uncertainty creates an unequitable burden, in part through the common performance of emotional labour. The potentiality of a wide range of GP responses may present a significant barrier; as with

Hal's or Jess's more general reluctance to see their GPs, non-binary people are primed to expect an environment within the clinic which does not understand them. In Jamie's case, their GP showed their lack of knowledge of this particular care pathway:

'The GP was like "I'm so pleased to see you, how many appointments have you had", meaning [GIC], and I looked at him and said "I'm on a six- to eight-month waiting list, which is one of the shortest in the country," and he didn't have a clue.' (Jamie, 24, interview)

The extensive waiting lists for GICs are well known within trans communities – as of spring 2019, waiting times for a first appointment across the English GICs was approximately two years, but has continued to grow. From Jamie's position, then, not being aware of a piece of information discursively coded as 'common knowledge' served to further undermine trust in the GP's ability to occupy the position of expert in relation to (trans) healthcare, which the doctor-patient relationship initialises and assumes. This example further emphasises the common need for trans patients to explain their healthcare requirements and experiences to under-equipped practitioners. Finn said:

My appointment with my GP where I asked for a referral was painful but ok – I had to do what felt like a tutorial in gender 101 with her, explain my identity, define different terms, and detail why I want hormone replacement therapy. I got asked a lot of questions that I don't at all see the relevance of – things about my sexuality, my relationships, my sex life. I answered them because I wanted to seem cooperative, but all the time I kept wanting to yell "THERE SHOULD BE TRAINING FOR THIS, WHY DO YOU NEED TO KNOW THIS, JUST REFER ME!" (Finn, 22, diary, emphasis original)

The most vulnerable non-binary people may therefore be even less likely to access referral, if they are unable to provide guidance to their GP due to being distressed by the interaction and unable to perform the associated emotional or instructional labour. Finn is clearly frustrated by a lack of adequate training on the topic of gender identity, such that the labour of educating practitioners can often fall on trans patients. This is problematic because whether or not such labour is (able to be) performed by the trans patient may change the outcome of the clinical interaction. In addition, the potential refusal of an uncertain GP to make a referral immediately serves to extend the length of time until a GIC appointment can be accessed. This may be a particular source of patient anxiety given the extensive waiting lists. Further, wide recognition of the potential for problematic interactions may result in trans people lowering their standards and expectations of healthcare – such that Finn still describes a 'painful' appointment as 'ok'. Trans people with negative experiences of medical care have extremely high rates of attempted suicide (Haas et al., 2014). This, together with 'poor experiences as common' being accepted as basic community knowledge may cause some individuals to downplay their negative health experiences when they feel that it 'could have been worse'. This relates back to how those reporting 'good' experiences – perhaps with this context better framed as 'not bad' – often framed themselves as 'lucky' (such as Ricky and Mark, discussed in Chapter 3).

In making such observations I do not infer that GPs actively demand training from their patients. However due to members of trans communities reporting smoother outcomes to each other when arriving prepared with NHS guidelines, or prepared to perform an educative role, there exists a sense within gender-diverse communities that such actions are advisable, if not necessary. David said:

> 'We hear lots of really great stories about really excited GPs, people come into the group with stories, "I told my GP I want a referral to the gender clinic, and they were like, this is so cool! I don't know what to do about this, I'm going to read all the books, can I google you?!" Sometimes you need to talk them off the ledge! It's quite bad, and the unintentional ignorance, and well-meaning ignorance, within the medical community towards trans issues, unless they are specifically working within gender identity that trying to bring in gender identity issues on top of that would probably make their heads explode.' (David, 31, interview)

This unpacks the important point that lack of experience or knowledge of trans healthcare does not necessarily mean that GPs are unwilling or insensitive. A practitioner's expression of desiring further information will have different ramifications, based on the symbolic interpretation of this by the patient. Mark's experience of seeking referral supports a general consensus that primary care practitioners are uncertain how to respond to patients outing themselves as trans and requesting referral. It is notable that rarely do these experiences involve specific mention of non-binary identity, likely due to appreciation by non-binary people that this could serve to result in a greater burden of education or further trouble their access to tertiary care. This would demonstrate the concept of 'strategic simplification' introduced in Chapter 4. Mark's account highlights his expectations regarding the presence of trans community, which was not met:

> 'The very first doctor I went to see ... well put it this way, my expectations going to see a doctor to speak about gender were ... I would talk about it, and I don't know, maybe they'd give me a leaflet or something, then perhaps they'd give me the details of a local support group and off I'd toddle with all my bits of paper, thinking "Ee, I've done something!" Didn't quite work out like that. Went to see a lovely doctor who freely admitted that she didn't have a clue. But having googled a few things – in front of me! – said she would find out. And actually, somebody finding out about stuff from an honest starting point I had no problem with. And actually, she was really good, and did get me my first referral. I didn't get my leaflet for a support group, because there wasn't one.' (Mark, 43, interview)

Mark went on to explain how this motivated him to create a local support group. This instance still illustrates that interactions with medical care can catalyse involvement with community. This may be because Mark felt ready, having taken the (medicalising) step that is discursively linked with legitimacy and security. This also highlights the additional problem that primary care practitioners may be ill-equipped to direct trans patients to additional support.

Lack of trans/non-binary education among clinicians, together with unfamiliarity with NHS policy and standards of care, are responsible for commonality in trans/non-binary patients perceiving excessive policing from GPs when attempting to be referred to a GIC. It is common for GPs to practice gatekeeping, only sending a referral letter if and when the trans patient has adequately performed their trans identity. Therefore, in order to manage (undertrained) primary care practitioners, non-binary people can utilise a binary narrative, explaining Jess's assertion that non-binary people can be 'forced into a binary gender'.

Participants also make points about perceptions of practitioners that cut across primary and specialist care:

'Everyone who I know who's trans has had really bad experiences with the medical community, both with trans-specific healthcare and general healthcare.' (Rachel, 28, interview)

This is a significant difference from other patients with specialist needs, who, while frustrated by gatekeeping practices or lack of ability to provide specialised care, are more satisfied with interactions with specialists (Kerr et al., 1999; Lewis et al., 2000). 'Coercive binarisation' and other causes of tension between GIC practitioners and non-binary service users will be further discussed in the next chapter.

Conclusion

The potential for non-binary identity to influence primary care experiences is multifaceted and extensive. Of particular note were the erasure of health complaints due to overemphasis of trans status, avoiding services due to negative experiences (or their anticipation), and concerns that raising gender with practitioners could negatively influence access to or experiences of other important healthcare services, particularly in relation to chronic illness. Further, treatment for unrelated medical conditions could alter the relationship had with dysphoria, or with gender itself. This could then feed back into social interactions that permeate all aspects of lived experience, raising many highly specific questions about trans healthcare intersections that have yet to receive any detailed academic attention. For example, how may disabilities influence GIC experiences, or, how do experiences of chronic health conditions shape or affect participation and involvement in different gender diverse communities, or vice versa (how does trans/non-binary status shape experience of disability/ chronic illness-oriented communities)? This would build on and relate to important empirical and theoretical work already conducted (for example, Kattari et al., 2017; Slater and Liddiard, 2018). While more work regarding trans and disability is warranted generally, non-binary-specific intersection with disability and illness would also be timely.

While participants reported positive and negative experiences, there was a universal sense that the non-binary *population* feels negatively about medical care, and broadly experiences that care negatively. This was particularly related to lack of awareness among staff (albeit with the caveat from some participants that staff could be well intentioned), leading to additional burdens of education and emotional labour for non-binary patients. Participants discussed important trends, such as the inappropriate over-emphasis of gender in medical contexts. Views of medical practice from non-patient perspectives (such as fellow staff member or trainer) provided additional insights into professional medical attitudes and knowledge when not performing the role of expert within the doctor-patient interaction.

The intersection of particular social phenomena highlighted serious problems with primary care experiences for non-binary people overall. Social processes of gendering are internalised uncritically within medical practice, and lack of specific or consistent training could leave medical and administrative staff unprepared and unaware of important and specific sensitivities relevant to non-binary identification, and transgender people more broadly. Being recognised by primary care practitioners as trans can depend on being read as such, which can be particularly difficult prior to, or without accessing gender-affirming medical treatment. In cases where trans status is recognised, this is uniformly within the gender binary, with no evidence shown of specific non-binary awareness. Indeed, those participants who were recognised as trans in primary care contexts did not press for a non-binary distinction, because of the difficulties with managing the situation as it already stood, thereby producing feelings of vulnerability.

Finally, administrative systems (including detail changes, feedback forms and secondary care information packs) all demonstrated important problems that affected how non-binary people went about or could negotiate existing medical practice. It is imperative to note that the heterogeneity of experiences in primary care will depend on factors such as whether an individual is deliberately presenting themselves in accordance with their birth assignment, whether they are regularly misgendered and how this affects them, whether they wish to access a GIC, and how much experience an individual has with negotiating clinical interactions since articulating their identity, if they have done so. Such factors also play an undeniable role in the negotiation of secondary/tertiary care at GICs, as the next chapter will explore.

Notes

[1]   For context of the asterisk after trans, see Tompkins (2014).

[2]   On 27 July 2015, the Conservative UK government launched a new select committee to examine the issue of transgender equality. A formal government response was published July 2016.

[3]   Not to be confused with intersex bodies – the non-binary body is non-binary by virtue of being the body of a non-binary-identified individual, rather than a reflection of specific physiological/anatomical arrangements.

[4]   Dildos also come in a dramatic range of sizes, rendering the comparison doubly unhelpful.

5 Myalgic encephalomyelitis, which, depending on the medical definitions used, may be used synonymously with CFS – chronic fatigue syndrome.
6 The 27-page version of the form can be viewed in full here (with the diagram described on page 9): www.whatdotheyknow.com/request/318902/response/785514/attach/4/1277%20APPENDIX%201%20First%20Assesment%20Questionnaire.pdf

6

A strong motivation to tick the boxes: non-binary perceptions and experiences of gender identity clinics

'I did once express how I was feeling confused about my gender ... and they promptly withdrew my diagnosis,' 'any sign of ambivalence is used as an excuse to delay your transition,' 'the fact that I confidently voiced uncertainty about my gender with the doctor meant that he didn't take my trans-ness seriously.' This particular issue was even more acute for those who did not define unequivocally as male or female. (Ellis et al., 2015: 12–13)

Introduction

There exists a wide body of literature addressing access to medical services for gender transition (for example, Dewey, 2008, 2013; Ellis et al., 2015; Pearce, 2018). This chapter addresses non-binary people's views and experiences of gender identity services. Echoing the opening of Chapter 5, this chapter first reports participant views of specialist gender-related care. This includes the perceptions of those non-binary participants who have yet to, or do not intend to, access a gender identity clinic (GIC), as well as views on how non-binary communities as a whole perceive such care in the UK. I follow by considering experiences had of both NHS-run GICs and private medical care.

Non-binary views of medical practice related to gender transition

There was a strong sense of agreement among participants that avoiding any mention of non-binary identification, or claiming a binary-oriented identity would be their best tactical option for obtaining access to gender-affirming treatments as quickly and easily as possible. This is supported in Chapter 3 by Frankie's discussion of their specialist physician explicitly positioning trans men and women as 'easier to treat' than non-binary trans people. In considering how they would communicate at their first GIC appointment, Jamie noted in their diary that 'I'm just gonna tell them I'm not female; that's not a lie.' They went on to say that:

> I haven't learned anything about their attitudes to non-binary people that would convince me to do differently than bend the truth to the max. (Jamie, 24, diary)

That Jamie '[had]n't learned anything different' reminds us of the common behaviour among trans people looking to access GICs to seek out as much information as possible about what to expect from their practitioners – using both official and community sources. Information from the wider community was a common base for participant scepticism with regards to GIC specialists (let alone GPs) being able to address their needs sensitively, broadly similar to views participants had of physician trans sensitivity in Chapter 5:

> 'I have had it expressed that some doctors are completely blind in this area, especially for transitioning, whilst others are more open to it, because they're just ... for some reason, especially with doctors who are in an area of transitioning, they don't even know anything about that. They always give the wrong gender, say the wrong things ... but they work in that area.' (Zesty, 22, interview)

Zesty indicates the concern that when specialist doctors working with gender make errors that are interpreted as a lack of cultural competence, trans people may then conclude that the specialist's 'expert status' does little to connect them to community and personal concepts of gender, which afford significant cultural capital. This is because of how sensitive and careful use of language is positioned as both fundamental and not particularly difficult by many trans/non-binary communities. Due to the now heavily interconnected nature of trans communities, many accounts of GICs are within intimate interpersonal networks, rather than from anonymous or unknown sources which may be deemed less reliable. Reports from trusted friends of inadequate experiences of healthcare are more likely to be taken seriously, and have a negative impact on the reputation of GICs among trans/non-binary communities. Community solidarity thus means scepticism of positive practice is more likely than scepticism of negative reports of doctors from other trans people, as with negative experiences of primary care discussed in the previous chapter.

Because of the sense within trans communities of both ignorance and insufficient nuance in the medical practice at GICs, the desire to perform the role of the good patient is explicit. In this context, the good patient is the individual who doesn't challenge well-established treatment precedent – matching that given to patients within the gender binary, and therefore clinical expectations of what constitutes appropriate trans care. Further, as in other medical contexts, patients must perform the sick role (in this case, fulfilling the practitioner's expectations of what it means to be gender dysphoric).

Stewart and Sullivan (1982: 1397) explain how in the context of many chronic illnesses:

> the entire illness behavior process appears to be characterized by definitional and role clarity, consensus and harmony. It is proposed that, in contrast, when physicians have difficulties diagnosing and treating an illness, as is the case in multiple sclerosis and many other chronic illnesses, the entire process is more problematic. The situation is less normatively controlled and as a result, social dissensus and disharmony are likely to occur.

Therefore, it is not simply *good* patient behaviour that individuals feel compelled to perform, but narratives that allow them to *be* positioned as patients. As already established, binary-oriented and non-binary trans identities are not chronic illnesses; the value in conceptual comparisons lie in how medical treatment pathways model and address them similarly.

Mark highlighted in his diary how this can lead to internal negotiations and performance of gender, which can lean towards gender stereotypes:

> The trouble is we soon learn how to jump through hoops. To be accepted as a trans man, one is expected (and not just by the medical/psychological people) to be a man. Be A Man. And it isn't just the outside world, either. Our internal censor tells us that if we aren't women, then there's only one alternative ... (Mark, 43, diary)

By switching from his typical handwriting to draw out the angular, capitalised and monolithic 'MAN' (Figure 13), Mark is highlighting

Figure 13: Stylised drawing of the word 'man', from Mark's diary

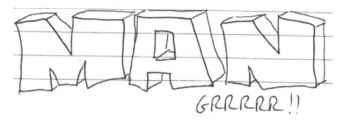

his view that in order to optimally 'jump through hoops', that is, to successfully fill gendered expectations, simply proclaiming one's gender identity with confidence and certainty is not enough. The stylisation highlights the difference between being a 'man' and being a 'MAN', the implication being that the latter embodies a desire to fulfil hegemonic masculinity (Connell, 1995). Such reflections from Mark resonate with Foucault's (1988) 'technologies of power', whereby individuals submit their conduct to a particular end, on the basis of an unequal dynamic with others. In other health contexts, such as the diagnosis of chronic fatigue syndrome (CFS), 'a diagnosis is a legitimacy awarded to those who are easily medicalized' (Clarke and James, 2003: 1389). In the context of gender, attaining such validation may be thought (or found) to be more likely if one constructs oneself to be as undeniable as possible through reproduction of hegemonic behaviour, producing a 'supernormal self' (Rinken, 2000) by exceeding the gendered demands made of gatekeepers.

It is also clear that Mark recognises such gendered policing as problematic. His method of highlighting his view (that hegemonic masculine presentation and attitudes are somewhat expected from people assigned female at birth) is presented humorously, with the literal 'GRRRRR!!' parodying and ridiculing rigid expectations of manhood. Importantly this is not simply directed at clinical practitioners, but also at wider society and 'our internal sensor'. Mark is here expressing his view that the synergy between not wanting to be read as how one was assigned at birth, together with doubt/lack of acceptance from others, and the corresponding insecurity and instability this can produce, can lead to overcompensation in order to legitimise oneself as trans. This can ironically then erase or diminish the specificity of non-binary identity.

While Mark's non-binary identification is such that he felt the desire for inclusion within this project, his view of accessing the GIC makes no mention of this, and was entirely in binary terms –

illustrating binarised gender enactment in the clinical context. An alternative possibility for some (see earlier discussion of the 'stepping stone process' in Chapter 4) is that non-binary identification may be 'arrived at' after medical transition has been successfully accessed. As also covered in Chapter 4, the positionality of non-binary as unstable, liminal or 'in-between' male and female (Wilson, 2002) means that the societal pressure to fit within the gender binary is an important differentiating point between binary-oriented and non-binary trans identity negotiation. Trans men and women can, in particular ways, still experience this; for example, those who have difficulty being viewed as their gender and are stigmatised as a result. However, the desire to be viewed as a man or a woman is inherently more intelligible, even while any non-cis modality can still be problematically excluded from male or female categories – the relegation of 'trans' to 'third gender' (Roen, 2002).

Jess builds on the suggestions that Mark makes regarding expectations (and evidence) of the clinic responding better to more normative articulations of gender:

'In order to get access to these medical treatments, you have to conform to cisnormative standards of beauty, you have to conform to cisnormative standards of masculinity and femininity. It often becomes a competition of who can fulfil these roles in the quickest and most attractive way. Even if you're a binary trans person that's how it works. Even if you're non-binary it becomes like a mini version of that. Who can perform these roles in those ways, but be with a kind of slight sense of edginess which is actually just like a very small socially acceptable dissent from that. But actually, there's no real dissent. Within the non-binary community, these kinds of norms, these kind of individualising competitive nature of the trans community which really does … which comes from above obviously, but really does undermine our community, our sense of solidarity, our ability to provide mutual aid and mutual support for each other.' (Jess, 26, interview)

The current medical system relies on the clinical judgement and assessment of secondary/tertiary care physicians, whereby a diagnosis of gender dysphoria must typically be ascertained before an individual can access hormones or surgeries. Jess's account emphasises her view that this system cannot and does not take account of how physicians can harbour socially constructed gender expectations and (conscious or unconscious) biases towards ratifying some experiences of gender over others. This can also be seen in the context of CFS, where the material evidence of the condition may be disputed. Subsequently, the culturally and temporally specific meanings of illness are reflected in practice, so as to discredit lived experiences, and disconfirm the possibility of diagnosis (Ware, 1992). Evidence of this can be found in the published work of senior clinicians, for example:

> These patients are very uncommon, and accordingly remain mysterious. They seem mostly to be female, and to have either a poor ability at (or perhaps a low interest in) interpersonal relationships. Certainly, there seems not to be any sexual motivation in what they seek. Patients of this sort nearly all had rather cold, schizoid, personalities. They have tended to lack humour. Two have been fluent in psychological-sounding jargon, yet were unable to draw abstract meaning from a common proverb. It is unclear whether there is benefit in acquiescing to these patients' requests. Certainly, the numbers are so small that there is not even a clinical impression of prognosis. It might perhaps be best to comply with the wishes of a group of four or five such patients (on the strict understanding that they accept that a good outcome can be in no way guaranteed), and then to declare a moratorium on all others until the first four or five have been followed up for at least 5 years. (Barrett, 2007: 43)

The book quoted here was authored by James Barrett, lead clinician and consultant psychiatrist at the Charing Cross GIC in London. Such views have hopefully evolved, as the visibility of non-binary people has increased extensively in the years since this stance was published. Two important points, however, must be made. First, any development in view will have been negotiated in relation to this earlier position, and thus discursively informed by its underlying beliefs and values. Second, the availability of Barrett's published account, easily accessible through the internet, means that non-binary people can (and do) take this as indicative of a *fundamentally* paternalistic and othering attitude.

Jess's point is that as long as roles must be fulfilled (to satisfy diagnostic criteria, and subsequently to access gender-affirming medical services), a hierarchy will form, favouring those able to fulfil the expectations and desires of physicians. While normative roles are performed by patients generally seeking all kinds of treatments, a non-binary identity inherently positions an individual as non-normative. The medical culture of normalisation therefore inherently and fundamentally disadvantages anyone with a non-binary identity seeking transition services. That said, changes in social and clinical norms regarding how trans people are conceptualised shows that 'boundaries of normality can be fluid' (Tishelman and Sachs, 1998: 48). The increasing challenge non-binary people have posed to medical models are encouraging professional shifts, such as how standards of care are conceptualised.

Jess's view that trans people need to conform to "cisnormative standards of masculinity and femininity" and the attitude captured by Dr Barrett's implicit distain at his patients being 'fluent in psychological-sounding jargon' are connected through a passage from Jamie:

> 'So, for example I read a horror story really, recently about someone online who'd seen a private gender clinic and been told "Oh you seem very feminine," (someone who identifies as male) "I think people have way too much access to information about being trans now, it confuses people...". This is all the stuff that I'm scared about [a doctor saying]. Pretty much every time I think about it, try to sleep actually, I start thinking "God, what will they ask me," how will I strike a balance between telling the truth and making sure they think I'm trans enough to get treatment? So that involves lying about, when I realised it, overemphasising some aspects of my past which I wouldn't emphasise that much, unless I knew that they kind of ticked legitimating boxes.' (Jamie, 24, interview)

Here we anecdotally see an unknown private physician, who specialises in gender identity services, voicing the opinion that "people have way too much access to information about being trans now". This is indicative of the view by some doctors that it is (and should be) the role of the physician to diagnose an individual's 'gender condition', and that their judgement is more reliable and authoritative than the patient's. This can be understood as doctors responding to a circumstance where 'symptoms' are unverifiable, and depend entirely on patient self-reporting. Such a reliance challenges the ubiquity of medical control, and can inspire mistrust in some clinicians. Illustrative of this, the self-reporting of pain by patients in prison who are diagnosed with cancer could be suspected by physicians to be exaggerated, as part of drug-seeking behaviour (Lin and Mathew, 2005).

A physician-dominated power dynamic is also implied by the view that there is a lack of transparency in GIC practices toward the gender-diverse population.

Jamie: 'Well nobody knows what the medical community
            thinks, and that's one of the major problems. We have
            no idea what they think of us.'
Ben: 'Do you think that scares people?'
J: 'Yes, very much. There's no transparency, we said before
            about waiting lists, there's no transparency about that,
            about what happens at appointments, or the attitudes
            of different clinics.' (Jamie, 24, interview)

This lack of transparency may be linked to notions in the medical community that such information would make it even easier for trans people to perform an expected gender role. When Dr Montgomery, former clinic director of Charing Cross GIC, was asked at the Third International Gender Dysphoria Conference his view on patients prepared to "do virtually anything" to access treatment, his response was "if you are prepared to lie to get it, then you can't expect the co-operation of psychiatrists" (Montgomery, 1994: no pagination). The age of this quotation means that it is important to recognise significant developments in practitioner attitudes over the subsequent decades. Such developments merit further study, as trans people's views of medical practice are significantly more studied than practitioner views of trans healthcare. However, this quotation does further contextualise the historical tension between trans patients and gatekeeping practitioners – that access to services must be 'earned by good behaviour'. Further, it illustrates how practitioners can deem it appropriate to essentially 'punish' 'dishonest' patients through the denial of service, rather than appreciating the social factors that produce patients who feel unable to be entirely candid. This is the employment of gatekeeping practices in retaliation for breach of one of Parsons' (1951) sick role criteria – that one is expected to cooperate passively with medical professionals to be granted sick role status.

Pig was very clear that while they would ideally like to access a GIC, they were unwilling so long as the system continued in its current form:

> With gender services, I would totally be up for talking
> to people about how I feel because I want it to be on
> record that I exist, however I don't wanna have to pay
> for the privilege of it, or have to be patronised by some
> middle-aged heterosexual wanker with a massive ego.
> (Pig, 30, diary)

As service users have no ability to select their (NHS) providers, and lack information about them (such that reviews are constantly sought within trans communities and on trans-oriented message boards), it is fair to say that the *perceived* risk of receiving such a clinician is high. This also raises a further element of GIC appointments – that non-binary individuals have the extra dimension of potentially feeling validated through 'being on record that they exist'. This could be experienced as exciting, or conversely as a burden or pressure. This is in addition to the potential to be disheartened by non-binary erasure within medical practice. Jess agreed with Pig's implication that GIC appointments do not necessarily centralise the non-binary service user's experience under current practices:

'I'm not really convinced that medical practitioners have non-binary people's interests at heart. And again, that's why people end up getting spewed out of the NHS system and de-transitioning, because they're forced into binary pathways. I think private doctors are much better at non-binary issues.' (Jess, 26, interview)

Jess articulates a view that there is a discrepancy between private and NHS transition-oriented care, whereby NHS guidelines may be more problematic than beneficial. This may be connected to the conceptual shift of patients to consumers (Hall and Schneider, 2008), and doctors as facilitators of choice rather than gatekeepers to resources. Private medical practice has been criticised in general for potentially engaging in excessive diagnoses and investigations in order to drive up costs, to the practitioner's benefit (Bhat, 1999). This does not translate well into the context of trans care however, as patients are not 'told what they need' by clinicians, but either make the requests directly, or undertake a process to ascertain what they feel they need (such as through a course of psychotherapy). While private healthcare is costly, it has the benefit of avoiding the extensive GIC waiting times that are a central point of criticism and frustration within trans and non-binary communities. More specifically to non-binary individuals, Jess's sense that private doctors are much better than NHS doctors may be due to feeling that binarised gendered performance is not (as) necessary in such contexts, as self-funding recontextualises the power relationship between service-user and clinician. The growth of private healthcare further underscores the discursive shift towards patients as consumers and doctors as facilitators of choice.

NHS guidelines require that gender dysphoria be 'persistent and well-documented' (NHS England, 2013: 15) for hormones to be prescribed. Jamie expressed anxiety at the idea of interacting with clinicians who may ask for information to determine the legitimacy of their desire for gender-affirming medical interventions. Jamie expounded on this in their diary:

> There is such a trust issue between the trans community and the medical community. No love lost. Everything I read tells me they're out to trip me up, to prove I don't really want it and haven't thought it through; that they start from a position of disbelief. (Jamie, 24, diary, emphasis original)

This trust issue that Jamie mentions can be conceptualised 'both ways'; gender-diverse communities are very wary of being pathologised or denied by medical gatekeepers. While there have been few explicit acknowledgements within the literature that some clinicians believe gender-diverse people to actively lie in assessment (Bailey, 2003),[1] clinical scepticism is now more subtle. For example, framing clinical assessment as 'the responsibility of ensuring that people recognize the decisions they are making' (Richards et al., 2014: 255), or to put it another way, the prevention of 'inappropriate' transition. While it is fair to argue in a context such as the NHS that this is a systematic requirement, the question of how health providers in different medico-legal contexts view concepts such as informed consent merits further study (Shuster, 2019).

> 'One of the reasons why NHS doctors are not very good on non-binary issues is because they're worried, basically, that non-binary people are confused, might detransition, might come back and sue, or that they don't understand these issues enough. So often it's a sense of covering their own backs really.' (Jess, 26, interview)

Through the hegemonic nature of cisnormativity, Jess argues that some practitioners see the purpose of gatekeeping (that is, assessment for eligibility) is to protect individuals from inappropriate treatment. This positions 'not requiring treatment' as the baseline for patient scrutiny and, in doing so, makes the assumption that denial of treatment (including delay through additional assessment) is the 'safer' route. Further, under such a system, experiences of regret from trans people may manifest in malpractice cases, such that it is in the doctor's personal interest to be conservative with treatment recommendation. This is despite the fact that existing clinical evidence presents miniscule detransition rates (Richards and Doyle, 2018). This helps contextualise why there is a modicum of consensus among participants on adjusting one's narrative to more neatly align with precedented, successful narratives. Alex discussed their potential plans for the future in their diary regarding GIC access, articulating some of their views:

> I'm thinking I might look into if I can earn enough to use some [money] on seeing a private gender clinic. The waiting list for NHS is currently 3 years on [clinic], and from what I've read online they don't have a great reputation for being helpful or easy to work with, especially if you're not someone who strongly and constantly projects the gender norms that they want. Which I probably won't – because even though I'd like to access testosterone, I do have a lot of 'feminine' interests ... and sometimes I still cross my legs when I sit – it's pretty comfortable. (Alex, 20, diary)

Alex here explicitly demonstrates their agreement with Jess's view that treatment access depends on the ability and willingness to fulfil expectations rooted in normativity rather than clinical necessity. They also illustrate a sense of being disciplined into the production of a supernormal self, seen through how Alex positions 'feminine interests' and 'crossing legs' when sitting as factors which, they feel, could place clinical doubt onto their claim of not being female. There was also the sense, as from Jess, that private treatment is preferable. The extent of Alex's sense that they would struggle to find the clinic 'helpful or easy to work with' may have extended into hypercorrection, as they indicate they feel even crossing their legs might affect a GIC appointment. While such scrutiny did demonstrably take place to this extent in the past (evidenced in Stoller, 1964), clinics are keen to explicitly state that judgements will not be made on factors such as clothing or sexuality (Nottinghamshire Healthcare NHS Foundation Trust, 2016).

There have been a large number of claims of improper or ignorant conduct towards trans service users in relation to gender, at the GIC level as well as in primary care. This was showcased by the 'TransDocFail' hashtag on Twitter in January 2013, where over a thousand people posted to highlight negative experiences. A follow-up survey was then created, prompting many of these individuals to formally report their experiences to the General Medical Council (GMC). This was summarised in a report by Helen Belcher (2014), one of the trans campaigners most centrally involved. The GMC indicated that they wished to investigate 39 of the 98 survey cases anonymously presented to them, with it particularly noteworthy that 63 per cent of complainants had not voiced dissatisfaction through any route before – implying that clinical feedback fails to reflect the number and extent of negative experiences. The reasons given for this included fear of treatment being withheld or withdrawn, lack of emotional resources to complain, and feeling intimidated.

This evidence suggests that trans/non-binary people not only adjust their behaviour to fit with the perceived expectations of GICs, but will also avoid challenging or disrupting physician behaviour they find unsatisfactory. Lack of clinical precedence of non-binary-specific narratives and overarching cultural unintelligibility are additional potential barriers to clinical access for non-binary services users. When asking Alex about their actions and intentions in the follow-up interview, they went into greater detail:

'I've been trying to see the gender identity service, and I am basically preparing to lie to them, because I know that they have certain criteria. You know, you have to have "socially transitioned" and changed your name, and all that nonsense, so I'm preparing to almost lie to get access to what I need to [...] I know from talking to people and reading people's experiences that doesn't tend to go down as well with the gender identity services. So, I've said I'm probably going to just be like "Yeah, no, I'm just a man, just a man, just give me hormones," because I think that's honestly going to be the easiest way to do it.' (Alex, 20, interview)

The most recent criteria that Alex could have been referencing were the Interim NHS England Gender Dysphoria Protocol and Service Guidelines 2013/14 (NHS England, 2013). However, the criteria for the prescription of hormone therapy do not formally require name change, or social transition. Indeed, the guidelines specifically state 'there is no requirement for the patient to have commenced a social role transition before a recommendation is made for hormone therapy' (NHS England, 2013: 15). Social role transition is required prior to accessing genital reassignment surgery. There is a significant lack of formal research regarding whether NHS physicians place demands on patients in addition to those within NHS protocols, prior to provision of treatment. Berg (1998) discusses how because protocols function as tools which restrict the autonomy of doctors' decision making in practice, they may be resisted as 'bureaucratic' or 'political'. The existence of protocols and good practice guidelines therefore do not necessarily guarantee the standardisation of medical practice.

This is significant in relation to non-binary gender identity, because of the lack of meaning behind 'living in the gender role that is congruent with the individual's gender identity' (NHS England, 2013: 19) when one considers non-binary people. While deconstruction of the concept of gender roles can allow this policy to be problematised even when applied to men and women, there is no obvious way it can be implemented in relation to non-binary people, as no 'non-binary gender role' is socially conceived. Further, current criteria indicate that GICs send a letter of recommendation to the service user's GP, who is ultimately responsible for the prescription of hormones. As the prescribing physician is ultimately held responsible, the potential for misgivings among primary care physicians is likely greater when confronted with any individual (whether binary or non-binary identified) if they present in a manner that challenges trans narratives that have been positioned as typical.

Frankie's personal development highlights how the demands made of trans people to fulfil gender roles may make it more difficult for individuals with particular gender (transgressive) expressions to access some treatments:

> 'I was never comfortable expressing masculinity from a male-bodied perspective. But since there have been changes going on, with my body, with my psychology and my frame of mind I've found it really, really comfortable to start exploring my masculinity.' (Frankie, 25, interview)

The vagueness around what a 'gender role' is in a clinical context, or how different practitioners may subjectively interpret this aspect of protocol, leaves feminine trans men (or AFAB non-binary people) or masculine trans women (or AMAB non-binary people) feeling insecure on whether they can fulfil the clinical criteria for genital surgery. There is little available evidence that suggests clinics are explicitly aware of, and sensitive to, trans people whose desired presentation, expression and identity exploration are not rooted in the 'opposite' position to the gender they were assigned at birth.

Minimisation or erasure of non-binary identification was not the only mode of resistance expressed, however. In Jamie's diary, they mentioned:

[Friend], who's been given a three-year wait at [clinic], is basically attempting to blackmail the NHS into giving him hormones sooner by writing a letter that says "I am going to start taking random hormones I've bought off the internet which will be super risky for me, so I am asking for a bridging prescription in accordance with your harm reduction protocol". If it works, he's going to put the text online for trans people everywhere to use, and we will break the NHS together or something... (Jamie, 24, diary)

This illustrates how many gender-diverse people have expert knowledge of the relevant guidelines and protocols, as this strategy utilises aspects of the good practice guidelines for the assessment and treatment of adults with gender dysphoria (Wylie et al., 2014). The guidelines indicate the necessity of medical practitioners to consider risks of harm in not prescribing hormones; highlighting the suggestion made by the World Professional Association for Transgender Health's (WPATH) Standards of Care (Coleman et al., 2012) of a 'bridging' hormone prescription while awaiting further assessment. The importance of community is also illustrated by the fact that the individual proposing this resistance to gatekeeping wishes to share the tactic with others, in order to challenge what is viewed as a problematic access restriction. Jamie's facetious positioning of this 'break[ing] the NHS' is not hostile to the NHS itself (on which the trans population is largely dependent). Rather, this phrasing can be interpreted as 'breaking' the barrier which removes agency regarding embodiment.

It is important to also note that views of GICs were not exclusively negative, which will be seen more extensively in accounts from those participants who have first-hand experience of GICs in the next section. However, positive comments were given, with caveats of the concerns already discussed.

'Some doctors are really quite good in championing the cause, I can think of John Dean, the head of NHS England's gender services, and he's pretty good really for non-binary stuff. He runs the Laurels, which is probably the best gender identity clinic for non-binary people. But he's definitely one extreme, and the vast majority of gender identity clinicians are either ambivalent or actively antagonistic towards non-binary people, in terms of either seeing it as a phase, or not really understanding it. I think there are huge problems with non-binary people who need to access healthcare who don't conform to people's binary ideas of what gender should be. So as a non-binary person, I would be still more likely to get healthcare if I presented wearing a dress, if I changed my name to a girl's name … I do have a girl's name, but if I did a whole bunch of stuff which is essentially conforming to a binary gender. I think what they're looking for is they're okay with you maybe presenting as non-binary if you essentially tick their boxes of what a binary trans person looks like with maybe a little bit of acceptable 'edginess'. But if you aren't interested in changing your name, if you aren't interested in adopting clothes associated with the 'opposite' gender I think you undergo quite a lot of heavy policing.' (Jess, 26, interview)

In comparison to Alex's earlier discussion of lived experience and name change, Jess articulates the view that heavy policing can be expected. This was on the basis of her experiences providing trans sensitivity training to medical staff, familiarity with medical policy, and, as with many of the participants of this research, extensive networks with many other members of gender-diverse communities. While some of the participants whose general views have been discussed have personal experience of accessing secondary and tertiary care in relation to gender, many do not (as also highlighted by some individual's discussions of their future intentions). The following section will focus on individual experiences of gender identity services, allowing for comparison and contrast with these more general articulations. Such a demarcation allows for difference to be identified between those who have interacted with tertiary care services directly, and those who have interacted only with the discourses about the services that exist within trans communities.

Non-binary service users' experiences of gender-affirming medical practice

Some of the participants in this study had a history of hormone prescriptions and/or having accessed gender-affirming surgical interventions. Because of the significant lengths of time accessing such medical services takes and the relatively small size of the sample, none of the participants accessed surgeries or hormones for the first time during the diary-keeping period. Even when access has proceeded smoothly for individuals, there was a recurrence of emphasis on having been 'lucky' or 'particularly fortunate' that this was the case. When asked his thoughts on the medical communities' interactions with trans people, Mark said:

'They're terribly scared of us! In my experience, which I appreciate isn't universal, I haven't had any horrendous ... you hear really awful stories, like, oh god ... but that hasn't happened to me, I've been fortunate.' (Mark, 43, interview)

Personal positive experiences, or at least the absence of significantly negative experiences, did not mean that individuals saw GICs as working unproblematically for the trans population overall. Ricky also highlights their awareness of disability intersection, as discussed in Chapter 5. While unable to explain the relative rapidity of their treatment access (which further emphasises the lack of transparency in GIC access, as raised by Jamie), Ricky did go into more detail about their case as being 'simplistic' from a clinical perspective. The explanation which Ricky gave of their experience being "surprisingly easy" was the ease with which their requests, from a physician's standpoint, could be conceived within the gender binary (matching that of a trans man).

That the clinic was very respectful of Ricky's pronouns, both in interpersonal interactions and when making notes on identity in writing, demonstrates both the capacity and precedent for clinical sensitivity in response to non-binary referrals. This runs contrary to the concerns of participants who had yet to attend, or did not wish to attend the GIC. This does not, however, allow an evaluation of the consistency across different clinics, or between the relative attitudes and approaches of individual clinicians. Indeed, clinical inconsistency is demonstrable, with Northamptonshire GIC having previously stated on their website:

At present this service is not commissioned to provide treatment for persons not identifying as male or female ... We would not decline a referral, as assessment and formulation of an individual's gender disorder may be more complicated than it appears to the referrer or indeed the service user. We may still be able to signpost an individual to another service.

However, this was brought to the attention of the NHS England Gender Task and Finish Group, who took this up with the trust as incorrect, resulting in removal of this text from the GIC website (Huxter, 2016). Given that there is a lack of empirical difference between the services offered to and accessed by binary-oriented and non-binary trans people, this raises the question of what is meant when the service positioned itself as 'not commissioned [to treat non-binary people]'. One potential explanation is that due to the ubiquity of the gender binary in the vast majority of discourses, commissioning documentation is likely to make no specific reference to the possibility of identification outside of the framework of male and female. The exclusion was in no way clinically justified, particularly emphasised by the willingness of other GICs to provide treatment for explicitly non-binary people.

Frankie had this dimension to add:

> My experience so far with gender identity clinics has been absolutely fine – other than the hideously long wait for appointments. (Frankie, 25, diary)

The significance of waiting times for GICs is an issue that affects all service users. NHS England (2016: 10) confirmed that 'people accessing gender identity services have a right under the NHS Constitution to be seen within 18 weeks of referral'. Freedom of information requests have been made to all UK gender identity services in order to establish how many patients have been referred to each, and their respective waiting times. For the period of August to October 2015, the average waiting times for a first appointment in England, Scotland and Northern Ireland were 44 weeks, 40 weeks and 11 weeks respectively, with a 38-week average (UK Trans Info, 2016). This has become significantly worse by 2020, with (for example) an average wait of 30 months for a first appointment at Leeds GIC (Leeds and York Partnership NHS Foundation Trust, 2020). This clearly demonstrates how the perceptions of long waiting times are empirically verified and not a simple case of an unfortunate minority, but the systemic inability of GICs in their current state to operate within the NHS constitution. While this is a problem across different medical services, it is particularly normalised, expected, and under-addressed within the context of GICs.

The examples in the previous section of participant concerns and plans of how to interact within the GIC are vindicated by the descriptions given of interactions by those who have already achieved access. While not highlighting problems with GIC staff, Mark did say:

> I get my treatment on the NHS, so there is a strong motivation to tick the boxes, say what I 'need' to say, and then bugger off to be who I wanna be. (Mark, 43, diary)

Mark clearly demarcates 'who he wants to be' from how he puts himself across in a clinical context – and given that, as a non-binary person, he has negotiated his healthcare without major incident, furthers the precedent to other non-binary people that engaging similarly can work. This, however, does not take into account the heterogeneity of the non-binary population. While obscuring or erasing non-binary identification for the sake of access is a viable tactic for some individuals, for others this may potentially cause distress similar to other experiences of being misgendered. While some participants (who used singular they as their pronoun) explicitly made mention that being misgendered with the gender they were assigned at birth is considerably more distressing, and that being misgendered as the 'opposite' to their assignment could even potentially feel positive, this cannot be generalised.

Frankie discussed their experiences of being out as non-binary within the GIC context, and how that was responded to in some detail:

> I've been reasonably open about my non-binary-ness from day 1 I think, though always used to talk about it within a binary framework. (Frankie, 25, diary)

This statement can be compared to Jess's critique that GICs will accept non-binary people "if you essentially tick their boxes of what a binary trans person looks like with maybe a little bit of acceptable 'edginess'". By utilising a 'binary framework' to articulate gender (such as through saying 'I feel more female than male') the doctor-patient interaction is managed, as Frankie has predicted, such that an articulation will be more readily accepted. While Frankie's self-conceptualisation shifted to feeling more binary than non-binary over the course of the research, Frankie wrote explanations of their more personal preferences for gender label use:

> I'm quite happy with the term 'non-binary', though not with 'genderqueer'. I'm not sure why this is, I'm just one of those anomalies who occupy a place in 'queer' communities but doesn't like the word 'queer' as a self-descriptor. For me I think it says both too much and not enough about my sexuality, regardless of whether it has the 'gender' prefix. Other I.D. descriptors I've used in the past and occasionally return to are 'androgyne' (too binary in foundation), 'transfeminine' (too feminine), 'demigirl' (sounds kind of inferior or 'less than'), and

very rarely 'woman' (WAY too complicated!). Recently I enjoy 'tomboi', 'bemme' (butch who's occasionally femme), 'hard femme', and 'riotgrrrl', and am finding progressively more solace weirdly in 'lesbian' and 'dyke'. (Frankie, 25, diary, emphasis original)

Such flexible and thorough explanation of feelings in relation to identity labels was not expressed as something any participants felt comfortable to vocalise in the context of the GIC. In relation to some participant narratives this could be thought to result from anxieties about delays to or denial of treatment. However, it is also important that while many binary-oriented and non-binary trans service users are confident regarding which services they need, others are not:

'When I first got to the GIC I didn't necessarily want to access hormones straight away, I didn't really know exactly what I wanted, I didn't identify as male and that was a problem. So yeah it [a course of therapy] was kind of suggested by one of the therapists and I was like "Yeah cool that sounds great, try that," and to be honest I feel like that was a really beneficial, positive experience. Compartmentalising a little bit, everything felt very muddled for a long time, and for a long time very hazy, it was very difficult to pinpoint what was going on, it helped me clarify things, compartmentalise, and work out how to move forward, it was brilliant. I can't thank [name] enough in a lot of ways. He was a really great person to do that with, just a really good counsellor.' (Frankie, 25, interview)

Frankie's account here points out how despite the general consensus of trans community voices highlighting the need for a reduction in gatekeeping practices and the need to challenge practitioners who operate from a position of 'trying to identify if the patient needs protecting from an inappropriate intervention', trans people also cannot be generalised to be expert patients, or necessarily self-assured of their needs. Correspondingly, this does not justify clinical behaviour that disempowers or disenfranchises non-binary people of their identities. Frankie noted that of one of their physicians (rather than their counsellor):

'The thing I've noticed most is pronouns. He uses the pronouns he thinks are appropriate, not that I think are appropriate. He originally used 'he', which was pretty uncomfortable. And I didn't really realise this actually until I went abroad, when I go abroad, because I've got an F on my passport, I usually take a couple of GIC letters just in case. Just anxiety really, just in case anyone stops me and questions it. When I recently went abroad, I rifled through some of my GIC letters and noticed this, I hadn't really noticed this before.' (Frankie, 25, interview)

This can be related back to Zesty's earlier point, that despite not having been to a clinic themselves, they felt "they always give the wrong gender, say the wrong things ... but they work in that area". Despite how Frankie said that their clinical experience had been "absolutely fine", they also said that "no one wants to be at that fucking clinic any more than they need to be". This shows that rather than universal clinical mistreatment, the alienation that trans people experience from the GIC, in practice, can be better understood and discussed in terms of the power dynamic between doctors and patients, which is structured by cisnormativity in practice – a lack of transparency, and inconsistency between different practitioners.

Leon provided information that demonstrated that, despite existing protocols being defended on the basis of the necessity of patient protection and the prevention of regrets, circumstances could arise where an individual with a history of hormone access could still be denied continued treatment. Leon explained how they first sought out treatment when living in the US. Accessing a low dose of testosterone within the US healthcare system proved to be straightforward for them; however, the prescription was recorded as being in relation to suffering from fatigue, which was also accurate. In advance of returning to the UK, and with a pre-existing awareness of the extensive waiting times to access a GIC, Leon's US physician provided them with a nine-month supply of testosterone. On explaining this situation at the primary care level, the GP refused to refill the testosterone prescription, with the justification that testosterone is unlicensed for the treatment of fatigue in the UK.

I've realised that my rationing of T (which is the prescription I brought over from the USA in September and I won't get an appointment with the GIC until at least May) is leading me back into muscle fatigue and exhaustion every month. Not sure what to do about that because I really don't want to talk to my GP about it and I can't speed up my appointment. (Leon, 34, diary)

There is a lack of recognition among the medical community that hormone prescriptions given to trans patients may also assist with symptoms of conditions separate from gender dysphoria (or a more general, unpathologised desire for hormonal transition). This is a reflection of the scenario recognised in Chapter 5, where medication for conditions unrelated to gender affected the experience of dysphoria, such as Rachel's opiate prescription. Because of the perception that transition-related care is a specialist area of medicine (which the existence of GICs for assessment purposes underscores), in conjunction with the ethical and legal responsibility taken by a clinician when making a prescription, many GPs feel ill-equipped to provide access to HRT without an explicit recommendation and guidance from a GIC (or suitably experienced and recognised private practitioner). In the 2012 trans mental health survey, 54 per cent of trans patients experienced a primary care practitioner telling them they did not know enough about a particular type of trans-related care to provide it (McNeil et al., 2012: 45). The report on transgender quality by the House of Commons Women and Equalities Committee (2016: 37) includes evidence from Dr James Barrett (lead clinician of Charing Cross GIC in London) where he stated 'a matter of serious day-to-day importance at a primary care level is the persistent refusal of some General Practitioners to even make referrals to gender identity clinics'. NHS England submitted evidence stating there was "Unwillingness by some general practitioners to prescribe and monitor hormone therapy" (House of Commons Women and Equalities Committee, 2016: 38).[2] Further, regarding the question of licensing – 'off-label' prescriptions are a fairly common phenomenon and can certainly be justified in and of themselves. Almost all HRT in the trans context is prescribed off-label, as the existence of trans is entirely erased from drug preparation information leaflets. This illustrates medical cisnormativity can be found in more esoteric contexts such as the pharmaceutical industry.

Some practitioners will give an NHS prescription on the basis of a private clinical assessment (which can save trans service users significant amounts of money through NHS prescription costs rather than private prescriptions, on top of assessment appointment fees). Leon needed to begin the process of GIC referral and access from the very beginning, despite two and a half years of taking testosterone, experiencing distress when they ran out. This indicates the necessity for healthcare practitioners (at the primary and secondary/tertiary care levels) to provide continued access to hormones when initially accessed internationally. Leon stated in their diary that 'I need the T to keep hold of a sense of legitimacy and strength.' The notion of legitimacy links back to the discourse of not feeling trans/legitimate enough without medical access. The legitimacy testosterone grants can be a source of strength (affecting emotional and mental health and wellbeing). Of course, it may also be the physiological relief from fatigue that the testosterone grants Leon – or even the literal 'source of strength', as testosterone stimulates muscular growth.

The same argument for hormone prescription, without, or prior to, GIC access may be applied in cases where individuals self-medicate through ordering hormones via the internet, though none of the participants in this study reported self-medicating. Primary care hormone access would allow for hormone levels to be properly monitored over time. Indeed, the 2013 good practice guidelines specify that 'A harm-reduction approach should be taken. Accordingly, hormones should not be stopped. A bridging prescription may be appropriate, and blood tests and health checks are undertaken to screen for contraindications' (Wylie et al., 2014: 183).

Such recommendations are reasonable because of the markedly low regret rates associated with accessing hormones or gender-affirming surgical interventions (Richards and Doyle, 2018). It is also worth noting that at least one major meta-analysis study of trans patient satisfaction, while recognising the low regret rate, also states that available evidence is very low quality (Murad et al., 2010). One participant did however give an important and nuanced account of regret, which was Ash:

> I do regret the phalloplasty. I can't orgasm anymore and I constantly smell of piss. It wasn't worth it. (Ash, 33, diary)

In considering Ash's experience, it is vital that this not be oversimplified, which requires contextualisation over Ash's lifecourse:

> 'When I went on the waiting list for breast surgery, I imagined that I wasn't actually going to have it. I did it because it was expected of me, and if I did everything that was expected of me, I'd get a prescription for testosterone. And I imagined I'd probably just go "Oh I changed my mind," and not having it done, and stop taking the testosterone, I thought a couple of years might be enough. But actually, I found it so interesting becoming more butch, and I was, my curiosity about what it would be like to actually pass as male just totally got the better of me, and I decided when they said "Here's a date," that I'd accept it.' (Ash, 33, interview)

From this account it can be seen that Ash's original intention was to never access mastectomy, but only a prescription for testosterone (and that, only for a while). That Ash changed their mind in direct relation to their experience of navigating the clinic and experiencing the changes that hormones produced can be compared with Frankie's account. Frankie found themself feeling 'more binary' after accessing hormones and made this link directly. Ash's identification remained non-binary; however, at the time of accessing mastectomy, Ash was embodying a masculine presentation and identification. They explained how through extensive exercise they experienced a large increase in muscle mass to the extent that their chest measurement was larger than pre-mastectomy. Ash articulated experiencing enjoyment in "embodying something completely different, watching the way the world reacted to me differently".

It is often assumed by doctors and the general public alike that gender identity (and corresponding embodiment) remains relatively static across the lifecourse. Yet for Ash, after a ten-year period they decided they wished to return to more feminine embodiment, though without a sense of regret in relation to their masculine time and embodiment. Initially they attempted further chest surgery to embody a 'non-binary chest', with an ambiguous structure that could be potentially read as pectorals or breasts, dependent on clothing choice. However, after negotiating this with their (private) surgeon, the result was unsatisfactory. Ash did not articulate this experience as particularly harmful however:

> 'But... it wasn't very effective. It just looked kind of like a lump which didn't look properly one way or another, it just looked like a fake lump thing in my chest, and I thought, "Okay if you're going to do it, do it properly," and I went back and said "Look, let's just do breasts," I've decided which way I want to go, and it took me a little while to feel comfortable with it, but the reaction of [sex work] clients just instantly changed. That suddenly they were happy with my chest, and I got more business, it paid for itself in a matter of weeks, honestly. And because it had made this huge positive difference to my life, I felt happier about it than I thought, and I really learned to like it in the end.' (Ash, 33, interview)

The intersection with Ash's profession as a sex worker is also significant here, as Ash experienced a significant economic improvement which synergised with their improved life quality overall, allowing them to 'learn to like it in the end'. This is a significantly different narrative to the earlier, NHS-accessed phalloplasty:

'I went in there going "Okay, I keep being offered this phalloplasty and you know maybe it would be nice, but I really have concerns about being able to enjoy sex, this is meant to make my sex life even better, and it's pretty bloody good to start with." So, I took some diagrams and said "Could we position things here," so from being the insertive partner I can really feel it, and we went through and it was a little more standard and he said yes. Then when I woke up, he said "We couldn't do exactly what you said anyway, so I did this instead." And it involved ... mutilating quite a lot. I was very unhappy, and he did his best to rectify the situation ... when I woke up, he'd not done what we agreed. And there's no way I could have known that in advance. There's no way I could have known, but if I had I wouldn't have done it.' (Ash, 33, interview)

From Ash's account, they were quite clear that they had not been coerced or manipulated. However, when asked if they thought there were ethical or legal ramifications to their surgeon's action, Ash explained that "It's a fairly specialist field of surgery, and if the guy who's the biggest specialist said 'I made a judgement call at the time, and that was correct,' everyone else believes that it's correct because he's the guy that knows." Further, Ash went on to say how the surgeon had clarified that "under normal circumstances the reports you get is this doesn't ruin things for people ... statistically I was unlucky". In comparing to earlier narratives of 'luckiness', this inspires a discourse of powerlessness – that whether one has a positive or negative outcome is difficult or impossible to influence. Here, Ash is internalising and accepting the surgeon's explanation that they were not 'normal circumstances', which discursively aligns with how non-binary clinical presentations are positioned as 'not the normal case'.

Ash did not say that they accept their surgeon made the best decision he could. Rather, they instead felt that attempting to challenge his authority would be fruitless because of his standing as 'expert'. Ultimately, trans patients (binary-oriented and non-binary) are dependent on the views and decision making of their clinicians, which is problematic given the lack of nuanced understanding that trans communities feel clinicians can have of trans particularity, which is sometimes evidenced through accounts some trans people give of interactions in healthcare settings (Pearce, 2018). Despite their self-assuredness in their genderqueer identification, it is particularly poignant that Ash said:

> 'If I hadn't had to present myself as a binary trans man in order to get some medical help, I wouldn't have then been repeatedly offered and guided in the direction of a phalloplasty. And the worst thing that's really happened to me ever wouldn't have happened to me, and that would've had a positive impact on my mental health if that hadn't happened.' (Ash, 33, interview)

This illustrates that discourses of inaccessibility and unequal treatment between non-binary and binary-oriented trans service users have a significant ethical impact in medical practice. In order to be mitigated, such discourses necessitate policy revision and revitalised training programmes that centralise gender-diverse voices. That Ash had even turned surgery down multiple times but kept being offered it, meant Ash "kept thinking maybe I am missing out on something, maybe my life would be better". There was also a critical queer community interaction to this experience, as Ash explained that at this time they were trying to date gay men, but experienced rejection – which may have been due to a phallocentricity among those Ash interacted with – "I thought it was that I hadn't had the surgery, and didn't have what they were looking for." This demonstrates how the immutability of gender as a binary within queer community and medical discourses can lead to multiple directions of pressure on non-binary individuals, to force themselves to pursue or perform embodiment and identity in undesirable (binarised) ways.

Conclusion

The chapter voiced that current guidelines force gender-diverse people to fulfil practitioner expectations, and to invariably compete with each other for limited NHS resources – as those deemed most in alignment with physician expectations of what being trans means will be conflated with possessing the greatest need. Further, keeping desired treatment within existing frameworks (such as only accessing surgery *following* hormones) also positions a non-binary service user as analogous with binary-oriented trans treatment access, and correspondingly straightforward to treat. Ease of experience in the clinic was often positioned as 'lucky' by participants, further reiterating the sense that GICs caused difficulty or distress more often than not. Even individuals reporting universally positive experiences criticised practices and practitioners in general terms. This can be understood when feedback is framed by the context of low expectations, and the multitudinous discourses of poor experience that mean negative incidences become 'part of the furniture'. One becomes 'lucky' not to have it worse, such that merely 'suboptimal' can be experienced as 'good', in relative terms.

Participants also raised the issues of lack of transparency in GIC decision making and processes, and a lack of trust between practitioners and service users. This was due to a sense that practitioners were concerned with maintaining a hierarchical power dynamic in relation to patients, and to protect themselves from potential malpractice lawsuits in the case of individuals regretting accessing treatments. The perceived bureaucracy of the NHS in the form of protocols, and most critically, long waiting lists, also meant that private healthcare could be (or could be viewed as) considerably easier to navigate, where affordable.

Among those who had already accessed gender-affirming medical services, there was an overall sense that their experiences had been positive. However, the fact that these participants still remained critical of GICs' service for the trans population overall was illustrative of additional complexity. There was a sense that experiences were made considerably easier by performing or emphasising (more) binary identification and/or expression. It was also made apparent that in resisting medical disempowerment of trans people, it is important not to then homogenise service users and risk universalising all those desiring treatment as expert patients.

This does not however mean that top-down power dynamics (which can involve direct disrespect of non-binary identification) cannot be addressed in practice. Leon's experiences of being denied testosterone in the UK following years of access in the US illustrated a lack of pragmatic ability to incorporate international synergy into NHS practice. Finally, Ash's case highlights how regretful outcomes may be further minimised, not by tightening the access to gender-affirming treatments, but by recognising a wider range of gendered possibilities as valid, such that gendered medical discourses are less likely to negatively affect patient choices.

In reflecting on this chapter, it is interesting to note differences between the views that participants had of GICs, depending on whether they had direct experience with them or not. Overall, participants communicated that there is a great deal of distrust and fear within the non-binary population of practice within GICs. This was explained with reference to a wide variety of points, including how practitioners' understanding of gender remains heavily biased towards the gender binary. This is a product not only of how fundamentally socially engrained the gender binary remains, but how lack of precedence/ visibility of non-binary patients discursively positions such individuals as 'non-standard'. In order to appease physician expectations, patients can feel the need to obscure or entirely erase their non-binary status through the construction of a supernormal binarised self, or through strategic omission so as to feel they are maximising their chances of accessing gender-affirming medical treatments. The conclusion of this work will address the themes in Chapters 3 to 6 so as to suggest recommendations in the light of this research.

Notes

[1] On page 172, Bailey (2003) quotes the clinician Maxine Peterson asserting that 'most gender patients lie', particularly citing sexual orientation as a factor that some patients feared may limit their access to surgery.

[2] The full evidence submitted can be read at: http://data.parliament.uk/ writtenevidence/committeeevidence.svc/evidencedocument/women-and-equalities-committee/transgender-equality/written/20376.pdf

Conclusion

I certainly believe that we can move toward de-regulating gender and still engage in important corrective practices like gender-based affirmative action. I am not arguing for a gender-blind society in which all people are similarly androgynous, but instead for a world in which diverse gender expressions and identities occur, but none are punished and membership in these categories is used less and less to distribute rights and privileges. (Spade, 2003: 29)

Summarising the narrative

This book has sought to address how non-binary gender identities are negotiated, within the contexts of heterogeneous queer communities and medical encounters. The academic foundations for this research were in both the sociology of health and illness, and transgender studies (most notably, an empirical sociology of trans experiences), with my approach to sense making and epistemological conceptualisation drawn from symbolic interactionism (Jackson and Scott, 2010) and social constructionism.

The research questions that were centralised within this study asked how non-binary people are involved with, and integrated into queer communities – where queer is used in a broad and holistic sense, near-synonymous with LGBTQ. If anything, my use of queer is sometimes broader, through the relevance of communities not specifically oriented with regard to gender or sexuality, but providing challenges to social norms, or opportunities to examine personal relationships with gender (and/or sexuality). In accessing such narratives over time through participant diaries, and also further reflections within semi-structured interviews, the data allows for broad consideration of how the increasing visibility of non-binary people within queer communities is accommodated (or not). From this, changes or necessary developments may be implied for the organisation of communities, and activism that is centralised within and around such communities. Further, this project's research questions examined how non-binary people negotiate access to and use medical services, at both the level of general, primary care for any ailment, and in the context of medical gender transition via a GIC. Concerns and social meaning ascribed to such interactions were considered broadly, such that discourses within the non-binary population were engaged with whether or not participants were currently seeking or accessing particular forms of medical care. The experiences and perceptions of the non-binary participants allowed for assessment of how current healthcare provisions for the non-binary population are viewed or experienced, and what implications this has for future provisions and potential methods of improvement.

A wide range of themes were identified through participant diaries and interviews, creating a framework for understanding negotiations and navigation of being non-binary. Non-binary functions as an umbrella term, including many individuals with disparate feelings about embodiment, presentation, and what interactions function to distress or validate. Yet, it must also be recognised that many individuals reject or resent an identity label that situates their gender in negative terms – essentially left as a vague 'not that'. Out of this have come community efforts to forge new language – perhaps most recognisable being the word *enby*, anecdotally originating from the phonetic similarity to the abbreviation 'NB'.[1]

Any essentialising answers to these research questions would be significantly limited. Trends were, however identifiable, allowing for original recognition of discursive influences, connecting interaction with medical service providers and queer communities. Some participants discussed their gender identities in terms of being static articulations of a third gender category. Others emphasised the fluidic nature of non-binary identification. Some were keen to acknowledge that, while they were happy with how they conceptualised their genders in the present moment, they accepted the possibility of having different feelings in the future (regarding making changes to embodiment, social presentation, or personal conceptualisation).

Gender-affirming medical services had been accessed by some participants. Others wanted to, and of this group, some were attempting to navigate such processes while others had not approached any service providers. Yet others did not desire to access medical services, and instead negotiated their non-binary identities in relation to their embodiment as it stands. Explicit cases were identified of participants whose self-conceptualisation had moved from binary-oriented trans to non-binary trans, or vice-versa. Participants could embrace a non-binary identity while at the same time preferring to use titles, pronouns and presentation unambiguously associated with the gender binary, which shaped how they were socially interpreted, and was assumed/subsumed into the gender binary by others.

Chapter 3 explored the theme of participants 'not feeling trans enough', which allowed for exploration of feelings of insecurity or instability in gender identity. How this manifested could vary, being indicative of internal self-doubt about the reality of one's status for some individuals, or for others be in relation to how they are viewed by others (including other trans community members, medical practitioners or more general social actors). A strong link could be seen between the discursive dominance of medical interventions in hegemonic trans narratives, and struggling for self-acceptance when not performing such narratives *even if* consciously recognising this as problematic. While participants frequently doubted themselves as 'not trans enough' by their own standards, or the standards they feared may be imposed on them, self-definition was sufficient for participants to accept others, highlighting a disjunction between how binarised norms of gender affected judgement of the self, versus judgement of others. In short, there was a sense that the non-binary people in this work upheld a politics of respect and recognition for gender pluralism, but could falter in affording themselves the same validation. I contend that this is produced through continual (sometimes subtle) discourses of 'trans as condition' (Pearce, 2018) in synergy with a broader social unintelligibility that can create increased difficulty in asserting self-knowledge.

Each individual's experiences were responsible for crystallising a particular understanding of trans (with variable absorption or resistance to hegemonic trans discourses, such as what medical and social transitions 'look like'). This crystallisation shapes their understanding of themselves and ultimately any conclusion about the relationship between their experience and their understanding of the 'non-binary' category/concept. Continual exposure to the percolating and often deconstructive discourses of transness shared around and blossoming out of communities render the relationship between identity and being quite malleable. As what one 'needs' to 'be' trans is increasingly deconstructed, I contest fewer and fewer people will feel they need to 'do' gender in any particular way to claim transness — if any property is essentialised, it is likely to be the sense that the individual's gender identity does not correspond to their birth assignation. For everything else, mileage may vary.

Historically precedented (particularly medicalised) narratives of trans-being could be resisted in how participants articulated their relationship with embodiment. Yet these might still be performed — such that criteria (such as gender dysphoria, or something less codified but associated, such as wearing or not wearing make-up) could still be fulfilled in order to justify being trans enough, both to themselves and to others. Rather than a clear distinction between a binary-oriented trans position as 'socially valid' and a non-binary position as 'socially unintelligible', the language a person uses (which may depend on who they're talking to, and that person's knowledge and political sympathy) can render this along a spectrum of sorts. That is, the non-binary person who articulates themselves in binary terms (for example, 'mostly female but a little bit male') and articulates a gender presentation that fulfils an expectation of 'in-betweenness' may find they can satisfy certain forms of enquiry more easily, by expressing a mode of non-binary being that is relatively accessible. This would be one example of strategic simplification, as conceptualised in Chapter 4. There is an intersectional complexity regarding how different non-binary people experience different forms of gendered privilege and vulnerability, however. While it might be harder for a non-binary person to be accepted as non-binary if their gender presentation is broadly concordant with expectations of their assignment at birth, they may also avoid certain forms of street harassment or risk of violence. I say intersectional because this illustrative example, among many other points of possible difference, is further shaped by race, class, disability and so on. The social difficulties in having to claim a gendered position in resistance, but ultimately not mirror-like 'opposition' to the assignment at birth can fuel problematic hierarchies of realness within trans communities (among both binary-oriented and non-binary trans people). Lack of intelligibility or awareness of non-binary identities within some trans communities could also lead to organisation or interactions that were uncomfortable or inaccessible for some non-binary people. Such accounts served to address non-binary involvement, and the extent or limitations of integration into some queer communities. However, these experiences only represented some of the highly heterogeneous examples of community organisation.

Chapter 4 engaged with themes that were collected under the broad idea of time. It was recognised how the passage of time, and the gradual process of identity reformulation – with particularly significant events, especially GIC interactions – correlated with adjustments to the relationship with gender identity. I proposed a visual model by which coming out processes, and the renegotiation of identity from binary-oriented to non-binary and vice versa may be visualised. The theme of identity as a stepping-stone process was related to the resources that participants may have access to in naming and processing their feelings with regard to gender (that could be age- or community-dependent). The theme of liminality provided a framework for conceptualising the potential fluidity or 'in-betweenness' of some non-binary articulations. This served to accommodate personal identity conceptualisations that demonstrated binary-oriented and non-binary overlap, which could be temporally or spatially situated, in terms of how identity was emphasised or expressed. It also rerenders medical transition as not necessarily having a 'fixed end point' (as binary-oriented gender transitions regularly assume), as gender cannot be assumed to be universally experienced as static over the lifecourse simply because desirous or deeply necessary medical interventions have been accessed. This allows for reconceptualisation of narratives and concerns about 'transition regret', which may be potentially used to delegitimise trans access to gender-affirming medical services.

Chapter 4 also covered the heterogeneity of non-binary involvement in queer communities, showing how a particular focus on trans people was not necessary for a politics of non-binary inclusion. Communities that might be particularly associated with defying normative practices or roles (such as Lolita fashion, or kink communities) or which challenge a gay/straight binary model of sexuality (notably bisexual communities) were explicitly highlighted as spaces appreciated by non-binary participants. This implies that the commonalities between non-binary gender identification and norm/role/binary disruption may equally be a source of affinity and support as communities oriented around trans status. Indeed, due to the breadth of possibility under the trans umbrella, tensions may readily manifest between different individuals. While a non-binary identity may currently be associated with anti-normative gender politics, having a binary-oriented trans identity cannot and does not indicate an individual's beliefs or approaches towards gender, with the potential to be conservative and reject queer or non-binary articulations, as was also expressed by participants who had observed this.

Participants shared a multiplicity of rich and nuanced views, and direct accounts of medical care. Experiences included examples where participants were impressed by service provider's efforts and sensitivity, or significantly distressed by their inadequacies. Accounts were divided into those not pertaining to medical-transition-related services in Chapter 5, and those which were, in Chapter 6. Of those which were not, many examples still related to 'gendered medicine' – services that inherently related to, differentiated or depended on the basis of how physiology is gendered, but through assumptions of concordance with the social categories of 'men' and 'women'.

In primary and secondary care contexts, non-binary patients were highly aware of how symbolic readings of them (or their genders) could affect their experiences of healthcare. While some participants were clearly determined that a change of gender be recognised on their medical records, it could be that removing association with the assignment at birth was of greater importance than whether this was changed to the 'other' binary category, or the pseudo-non-binary option of 'unspecified' – in terms of distress mitigation. Participants expressed that anxiety over the perceived likelihood of lack of understanding or potential stigma in primary care contexts could delay them from scheduling important medical checks or condition management, or even result in total avoidance of medical care.

Problems could be encountered with medical practice prior to doctor-patient interactions. Administrative processes, documentation and exchanges with clerical staff could erase identities. Such difficulties could require significant patient (emotional and/or educational) labour in order to be recognised, or place an individual into a vulnerable state prior to a medical appointment. Participants expressed how trans identification could be inappropriately conflated with, or distract from, independent health issues. This point reiterates how some social and medical experiences are similarly experienced by binary-oriented and non-binary trans people; however, appreciation of specificity may produce necessarily different approaches for improving a given problematic interaction. Valuably, some participants described interactions with healthcare providers in contexts where they were not a patient, but a colleague or trainer. This raised issues such as the potential for problematic or offensive behaviour from other staff when trans or non-binary patients are not within earshot, evidencing a cisnormative culture within medical practice. Such a culture codifies gender diverse people as a 'patient subgroup', ossifying trans/non-binary status as 'condition' rather than a broader facet of being – erasing recognition of their existence in non-patient contexts, particularly as colleagues.

Further, particular barriers were expressed for non-binary people with chronic health conditions or disabilities. In some cases, extensive interaction with health services unrelated to gender identity primed individuals to expect problems when seeking assistance. Participants could be concerned that raising a discussion of gender identity would risk disrupting treatment for their other conditions, positioning such an action as unacceptably hazardous for them. Highly specific interactions also recognised the potential for interaction between conditions and transness – through medical interventions (such as Rachel's experience of taking opiates and the impact in mitigating dysphoria that was otherwise not being professionally supported) or social navigations (such as Jess's sometimes-strategic use of her walking stick).

The referral process, whereby primary care practitioners formally have a patient placed on a waiting list for an appointment with a particular GIC, was of significance to many participants who wished to access a medical transition but had not yet done so. Examples were given where GPs would attempt to assess participants prior to referral, which in addition to being contrary to best practice guidelines, inadvertently reinforces the binary gender hegemony that many medical practitioners uncritically reify in patient interactions.

The theme of obscuring or omitting non-binary identification carried into tertiary care (GIC) contexts, was explored in Chapter 6. It is notable, however, that while participants with positive experiences in their receipt of gender transition-related care did not want to imply that services were without (systemic) faults, they did also discuss the positive aspects. Those who had not accessed clinics directly were highly concerned with the negative experiences that were discussed within community contexts. There has been extensively problematic treatment of trans people in clinical contexts, particularly historically under now antiquated modes of practice. Lack of transparency regarding methods of assessment and medical decision making means that shared community knowledge nucleates from accounts by those trans individuals who pass through GICs. As all service users wish to conclude their interactions with the GIC as quickly and easily as possible, there is significant focus on performing those gendered roles that are judged to best satisfy clinicians. This can be significantly more difficult when an individual is openly non-binary, due to comparative lack of clinical precedent, particularly if they are desirous of interventions that transgress historic pathway expectations. This is slowly changing, with it being increasingly possible, for example, to access mastectomy prior to or without HRT, to access low-dose HRT, or to access hormone blockers (with calcium/vitamin D supplementation to protect bone health) for those who want a more 'neutral' hormone profile. Developments and reconceptualisations of medical possibility have seen more 'radical' possibilities legitimised in medical contexts elsewhere (such as the US). Known examples include the provision of vaginoplasty while keeping the penis (Vincent, 2019) and the agreement of a surgeon to perform vaginoplasty in a context where the patient was private about their relationship with gender in their professional life and continued to present as a (cis) man.[2] Restrictions concerning medical interventions (that aren't dictated by what is ultimately possible) may, in surgical contexts, be due to a lack of practitioners with the training or experience in certain newly developed techniques. In cases such as the latter example, restrictions of patient autonomy relate to clinical responsibility in the context of UK healthcare provision. This ultimately relates to the differential interpretations of what constitutes an 'informed consent' model of healthcare (Deutsch, 2012; Cavanaugh et al., 2016).

Some tertiary care practitioners did not seem to engage with non-binary articulations of gender identity as being equally valid to binary-oriented trans identities. Concerns with non-binary patients being 'more difficult to treat' could be grounded in a reliance on clinical precedent rather than holistic engagement with the individual. In addition, such practice risks assuming that desired medical interventions for non-binary people are necessarily able to be demarcated from binary-oriented trans-being, when no particular medical treatment (or lack thereof) is essentialised to, or defines, binary-oriented or non-binary identification. While differences may be identified when studying *populations* in comparison (Burgwal et al., 2019; Rimes et al., 2019), this is fundamentally different from situating binary-oriented precedent as the yardstick by which non-binary requests for medical intervention are measured.

Insecurity related to not being trans enough was observed in relation to all three subdivisions of interaction that are conceived within a symbolic interactionism. These are: not feeling trans enough by one's own standards (intrapsychic interactions); anxiety over being seen as trans enough by other community members (interpersonal interactions); and being considered to be trans enough to access services or processes dependent on trans status (cultural, or structural, interactions). The latter is most obviously medical interventions, but also has a legal remit – for instance, whether an individual feels protected by the characteristic of gender reassignment within the Equality Act 2010 (as of early 2020, specific discrimination on the basis of non-binary status has not been tested within the UK courts), or whether one feels able to navigate the process of obtaining a gender recognition certificate (albeit within the binary) via the Gender Recognition Act 2004. Further, the anxiety over the uncertainty of a 'smooth transition' means that communities are likely to focus on negative narratives of healthcare over positive ones, in order to 'be prepared' for clinicians with particular reputations. Trans expert patienthood (supported by interactions and resources shared within trans communities) was obtained by participants in order to manage practitioner expectations and the medical gaze. However, performances of gender not only served to fit into the role of a 'good patient', but necessarily as patient *at all*. The necessity of a distress-dependent experience, oriented around embodied dysphoria in order to be deemed 'diagnosable' by physicians limits the narratives that can be safely explored in a clinical context, due to the anxieties surrounding the potentiality of service provision denial.

Research recommendations

One of the most fundamental recommendations for medical practice that can be made is inspired by those communities that non-binary people expressed affinity with, such as bisexual and kink communities. Such spaces were sensitive and reflexive to gender plurality, and tended to construct language and space to be more fully inclusive. Gendered assumptions rooted in cisnormativity need first of all to be recognised, and then challenged within medical practice. Much of this may be done through the provision of training to both medical students, and existent medical staff and administrators. This already occurs, but with great inconsistency, and is dependent on the proactivity of individuals with decision-making powers in local contexts rather than as a consistent, universalised dimension of professional training. The significance of language in erasing non-binary genders and potentially triggering dysphoria is such that the use of gender-neutral forms of address ('good morning', rather than 'good morning, sir', for example) when individual preferences/needs are *unknown* – and not assumed from gender presentation, name and so on – should be normalised in practice towards all patients. This would also benefit binary-oriented trans people who are not out, who are pre-transition, or who are commonly misgendered, and cis people who may also have complex and personal reasons to avoid aspects of gendered language or bodily assumptions. Administrators should be clear on how to (and that they can) change a patient's gender marker to 'unspecified', with health professionals being aware of the contexts in which this may have interplay with experiences of care (such as gender marker-dependent screening notifications for breast, bowel and/or cervical cancer, and abdominal aortic aneurism).

How gendered medicine is practised may be similarly adjusted at the administrative level to improve preventative health screening for gender-diverse people, an example being who receive letters reminding of the necessity of smear tests. At present, this relies on the flawed conflation of the categories 'people with an F gender marker on medical records' and 'people with cervixes'. Changing this would benefit more of the population than gender-diverse people, such as people with known intersex conditions, and cis women who have had mastectomies or hysterectomies. Systemic changes would also need to be accompanied by standardisation of training on trans healthcare within medical and nursing degrees, as well as staff training for administrative roles. Such interventions have lagged behind the still-modest but precedented production of continual professional development (CPD) accredited training, such as e-learning hosted by the Royal College of General Practitioners, and the Pride in Practice initiative managed by the LGBT Foundation in Greater Manchester. Such actions would render trans identities as more intelligible generally, and equip staff in delivering medical practice that would be clipped of gendered assumptions.

With regards to gender-affirming medical services, good practice guidelines stipulate that 'patients are presumed, unless proven otherwise, capable of consenting to treatment' (Wylie et al., 2014: 169). The fact that individuals referred to GICs are required to undergo a process of scrutiny prior to being able to access HRT illustrates how patient competence and willingness are insufficient under current (NHS) provision. A system of gatekeeping assessment[3] attempts justification by appealing to the need for accountability of taxpayer-funded NHS resources, and the ultimate legal responsibility of the clinical provider, which I will address in turn. Regarding costing concerns, HRT is ultimately not an expensive set of medications for the healthcare system. Significant administrative and practice costs would also be saved in the elimination of psy-oriented assessment as a specialist prerequisite. Timely receipt of gender-affirming medical interventions would also likely reduce the draw on mental health services through the lessening of dysphoria-related depression and anxiety, and likely reduce (the very high rate of) attempted suicides. It is worth noting that concerns over care with public funds tend not to be applied proportionately, with any rise in HRT costs being orders of magnitude less significant than tax evasion and avoidance, the Trident nuclear programme, or the projected fiscal damage caused by Brexit, for example. Further, with waiting lists what they are we must be clear: the only reason the NHS is not needing to account for the costs of more patients accessing HRT is because of the GICs acting as bottlenecks, and patients are being denied access due to waiting times that come at horrendous individual suffering. Ultimately, I also argue that because it is ethically necessary to move towards an informed consent model of trans healthcare, practitioners should not bear the same degree of ultimate responsibility should they be following best practice guidance and following the wishes of a fully informed service user, capable of consent. There is a question of balance of course, as patients still need to be protected from potential malpractice, with power differentials creating barriers to challenging medical judgement after the fact.

Gender dysphoria (or indeed, any wider set of conceptualisations that may motivate an individual to access gender-affirming medical interventions) depends on self-reporting. This is not unusual in medical contexts, with perhaps the most obvious example being when reporting the severity of pain. Nor is trans health unique in being a non-pathological circumstance that necessitates specific care – pregnancy being an obvious example. Yet, the particularity of trans healthcare might be unique in bringing these factors together – non-pathological status (Richards et al., 2015), 'un-testability', but total professional recognition of the necessity of funding and intervention – both improving lives, and sometimes saving them. I particularly draw attention to HRT because of the relative simplicity of its administration, and because a significant proportion of gender-diverse people are highly confident of, and consistent in, their desire for HRT, compared to a larger number of cases of reticence/complexity regarding surgical desire. Even were it not the case that culturally constructed and maintained binary norms of gender influence tertiary clinical practice, such that non-binary patients are potentially coded as 'more difficult' or 'more complicated', it is problematic that any transgender transition-oriented care does not grant autonomy over how an individual wishes to negotiate their embodiment. Further, this is in a context whereby gender identity services are beginning to collapse under the strain of demand with waiting lists almost universally multiple-years long, without corresponding growth in resource allocation or staffing.

Given the constraints on NHS budgeting, there is clearly a finite amount of funding available to assist GIC patients. Therefore, there are at least two critical factors indicating that the current healthcare system results in patients being positioned as competing for resources. First, there is the necessity for patients to fulfil imperfect diagnostic protocols and subjective expectations of individual clinicians. Second, resource limitations, partially a result of more general underfunding of the NHS (Campbell, 2015; Pym, 2016), inefficiencies (Niemietz, 2016), under-recognition of the importance of gender-affirming medical intervention (Prescott, 2019), and the rapid growth of the trans population trying to access services (Lyons, 2016). For as long as the patient population continues to grow without proportional resource allocation, tertiary care providers will only be equipped to facilitate a limited number of transitions over a given period of time. Whether individual waiting times are triaged (at the discretion of practitioners) is broadly unknown, due to lack of transparency concerning clinical practices and management. There is a need for the assumptions regarding non-binary people being viewed as 'less certain', or as experiencing less significant dysphoria than binary people, to be explicitly addressed in clinical training. A vital dimension which would benefit from more research is clinician experiences of care provision. This could also include how to support clinicians to engage with and manage criticism from gender-diverse people on the one hand, and anti-trans activists on the other. There is a challenge for clinicians in recognising that being well-intentioned does not eliminate the possibility of causing a patient distress (or even harm), either through their approach/attitude or their management of the tension between gender-diverse people and healthcare systems. Social conditions create an environment that may leave clinicians feeling defensive, which needs accounting for in any training that incorporates the nuances of gender-diverse criticism of healthcare practice and systems.

Gender-diverse people's hormone access equivalence could be established and significant relief granted on GIC resources through the allowance of hormone access without the necessity of GIC assessment. In the context of hormone provision, a primary care practitioner could review expected physiological changes, and any associated health risks. Blood tests are taken in order to establish initial hormone levels; risks and expectations are discussed to establish informed consent and patient-centred care. There is already significant movement in this direction, with a key example being the set-up of local gender teams in each health board region of NHS Wales to ensure equality of HRT access and to assist GPs in the direct provision of HRT. A pilot scheme in Greater Manchester also aims to trial a new delivery model for gender-related care.[4]

By centralising patient agency, the deference to gender specialists (who do not have specific or particular training in how they respond to service-user reports of being trans, and whose expert status is defended/obtained on the basis of accumulated experience in undertaking assessment) is largely reduced. Of course, endocrinological and surgical expertise are still hugely important for consultation where necessary. Correspondingly, by only requiring GIC referral for surgical assessment, waiting lists would be significantly reduced. The fact that patients already require primary care appointments to obtain referrals, receive hormone prescriptions and monitoring from primary care practitioners on the recommendation of GICs, means no additional burden would be placed on the primary care context. The removal of an assessment-oriented framework (that currently requires a minimum of two appointments at a GIC prior to diagnosis and HRT recommendation) would save on costs for the NHS, and for individual patients who often must travel far and/or stay overnight for appointments (as of 2020 there were seven adult GICs in England, two functioning clinics in Scotland, a new clinic in Wales, and one in Northern Ireland). Further, the eighth edition of the WPATH *Standards of Care* is in production as of mid-2020, which is expected to see yet a further shift towards reducing psychological or psychiatric assessment. This edition of the guidelines will also introduce new chapters, including one specifically addressing provision of care for non-binary people.

Recommendations for community organisations are inevitably less structured. Difficulty may be experienced by organisers who encounter tensions between group members, especially when feeling unequipped to diffuse or police such interactions, and indeed, the total elimination of intragroup tensions is not feasible. Being mindful of the potential harm of self-validation through comparison to (less 'successful') others, and of the risks in assuming the homogeneity of trans identities (such as wishing for surgeries) would likely improve community experiences for non-binary people. This may be attained through increased communication between community leaders and organisers, which is significantly easier via digital community spaces such as Facebook and Tumblr. Further research would be beneficial regarding the boundaries and impacts of the label 'trans' for non-binary people, and how ossifying notions of what constitute 'transness' can affect self-conceptualisation and interpersonal relationships. Work by the Scottish Trans Alliance (Valentine, 2016c) showed 15 per cent of non-binary people did not identify as trans, and 20 per cent were unsure. This significant minority should not be erased through the admittedly convenient framing of 'binary and non-binary trans'.

Cautions, limitations and future directions

Recognition that this research has served to offer a snapshot of non-binary experiences and views within a particular cultural context and at a particular time is important when considering this work's impact. Formal policy, medical training practices, the cultural intelligibility of non-binary identities, and community norms and practices continue to develop and shift. Recognition of non-binary narratives is essential for queer communities and medical practice to be inclusive of gender plurality – which must be through dismantling structural and systemic barriers.

Problematising cisnormative cultural practices, whereby all individuals are assumed to be cisgender by default – and correspondingly therefore, that trans individuals may be necessarily visibly identified – is a macrosociological observation. However, examples within the data drew attention to individual acts of practitioner and community member insensitivity. I argue that this is illustrative of widespread issues on the basis of social context in addition to participant accounts, but this is not generalisable to *all* healthcare practitioners, or to queer community members who are not non-binary. While it is undeniable that there are individuals who engage in discriminatory and offensive behaviours, the significance of the lack of awareness of non-binary gender identities, in particular, and the ability for well-meaning individuals to engage in or perpetuate problematic behaviours cannot be overstated. At the level of the individual, education initiatives that challenge simplistic and assumption-oriented judgement making in social interaction would have a marked impact, yet the structural constraints of gatekeeper-oriented healthcare would still remain. From this research, it is not possible to make definitive inferences as to whether the negative views of medical care within the non-binary population are entirely rooted in examples of problematic practice. These certainly occur to a disproportionate standard, as supported by existent transgender health studies (Bockting et al., 2004; Dewey, 2008; Bauer et al., 2009; Bradshaw and Ryan, 2012; McNeil et al., 2012; Kosenko et al., 2013; Hagen and Galupo, 2014; Ellis et al., 2015). However, aspects such as the potential for individuals to be sensitised by communities to expect poor experiences, or for non-binary people to articulate poor experiences as acceptable because of exceeding especially low expectations, require more detailed attention.

With regards to the demographics of the sample, as discussed in Chapter 2, all except for one participant were white; therefore, the sample did not reflect the experiences of gender diversity that may be found among different ethnicities. All but one participant had attained (or were in the process of earning) a degree. Extrapolating on the basis of educational attainment and the overall contexts that researcher-participant interactions have allowed, I therefore suggest that the sample is skewed towards middle-class representation. While Harrison et al. (2012) evidence that non-binary people (in their North American sample) had above-average educational attainment, my sample is nonetheless not necessarily broadly comparable to the overall UK population. This is likely a result of some of the avenues used in the recruitment process, such as university-based LGBTQ societies, and the potential for a homogenised sample as a result of snowball sampling.

Limitations associated with the methods used in this research were also articulated in Chapter 2. However, the extensive labour involved in diary keeping was certainly apparent by seven out of 25 original participants withdrawing from the project, many due to feeling unable to commit to the extent of participation required. Further, the number of participants with prior diary-keeping experience suggests that the method may have played some role in self-selection; non-writers may have found the project less accessible – and become less accessible themselves due to this. While one goal of the diaries was to access more routine aspects of non-binary life and experience, the interviews emphasised more demarcated, unique happenings such that relatively recent interactions were possibly overemphasised, particularly if compared to the roles of queer community or medical practice in participants' lives prior to the diary keeping exercise.

This study did not target any particular sites of medical practice, GICs or community organisations for scrutiny of their interactions with non-binary people. Therefore, recommendations cannot be made in relation to any specific organisation's current policies, as it is unknown to what extent participant experiences would necessarily be representative for a given set of service users. However, the data does allow for a more general approach to service improvement, which if borne in mind could see policy becoming more standardised and care become more efficient and holistic.

With regards to future research directions, an enormous amount of possibility remains open for research in relation to gender beyond the binary. Lack of quantitative data on non-binary people[5] beyond very rudimentary extrapolated estimations from community members renders population studies difficult. Adjustment of census questions so as to be able to record people identifying outside of the gender binary, and also with a trans identification more generally, would open a wide range of research possibilities. Intersections between non-binary gender identities and different forms of social inequality would also provide excellent sites for academic scrutiny. Of particular importance would be detailed work on disabled and chronically unwell gender-diverse people, and consideration of the often-underacknowledged older (50+) non-binary population. The organisation of trans-specific pride events speaks to the emergence of politically galvanised communities; research into the conceptualisation of activist identities (and how this cuts across different political issues such as refugee rights, prison abolition and climate change) would be of great value. In the contexts of other disciplines, there is a significant absence of culturally competent and sensitive medical research considering trans health experiences that transgress historical precedent (such as the impact of lower doses of hormones in different bodies at different ages, for example).

We're here, we're genderqueer, get used to it!

In summary, the integration of non-binary individuals into queer communities is most apparent in the specific contexts of trans communities, more so than broader LGBTQ examples. Some participants indeed highlighted cis gay men as a group more likely to express intolerance or lack of understanding of non-binary identities, in a manner which may alienate. There were multiple examples of non-binary involvement and integration with various sexuality or gender-related communities, but with the commonly shared trait among community members of being particularly accepting of differences in gender identity and expression.

The negotiation of existing medical practices is currently fraught with anxieties and potential difficulties for non-binary individuals, perhaps most centrally a lack of intelligibility among the majority of healthcare practitioners. The specific circumstances of care may necessitate different forms of educational or policy intervention in order to see improvement. While experiences were certainly not universally negative, the recent cultural emergence of non-binary identities means that health services need to respond quickly in order to avoid compounding risk of harm to this significant minority group of service users.

For queer community organisations, non-binary identity emergence implies that recognising the necessity of resisting the uncritical incorporation of gendered norms into community practices is required for pluralistic, inclusive and inviting spaces and events. It can be argued that the relative social disempowerment of cisgender gay men and lesbian women (when compared to the trans population) has considerably lessened since the new millennium (McCormack, 2013). This, together with the fracturing of queer solidarity along the lines drawn through identity politics can mean that non-binary identities risk being stigmatised. This may nucleate through homonormative ideals, or depoliticised and over-simplistic internalisations of gender by some gender-diverse people. That said, there are also examples of non-binary individuals being celebrated and embraced by communities, and also the creation of increasingly specific and nuanced groups and networks, particularly in synergy with digital technologies.

In the context of trans/queer healthcare, non-binary gender identities suggest that discourses are shifting, to render the maintenance of arbitrarily rooted and uncritical gender roles within medical practice increasingly untenable. Non-binary identities highlight the importance for *all* medical practitioners to have an appreciation of the potential problems and limitations of gendered assumptions in any social interaction, particularly in the prospective situation of engaging with a vulnerable individual. Non-binary gender identities also provide a valuable avenue for the reinterpretation of many narratives of de-transition. This further suggests that holistic trans healthcare is not possible without full acknowledgement of the possibilities of gender plurality, particularly as an individual's needs change over time.

A final observation: I have noted through my experience of queer communities that if one considers LGB people, binary-oriented trans people, and non-binary people, the speculative bell-curves that represent their respective distributions across the political spectrum are shifted more and more to the left. Why is this? A simple answer might be that marginalisation (or at least, a personal investment in challenging a particular form of social injustice) increases criticality of the inequalities produced through capitalism and the exertion of power by the state. My tentative hypothesis is that undergoing a process of identity negotiation that involves challenging the monolithic and ubiquitous discourse of the gender binary opens up the possibility for individuals of challenging *other* seemingly-inevitable social systems that are sites of inequality. This especially nucleates the recognition of intersectional consideration of social and material injustices. The interconnectedness of macrosocial problems is being increasingly signposted in popular left-wing discourse, with Oliver Thorne of popular YouTube channel Philosophy Tube saying "If you campaign for migrant's freedom of movement, you are fighting climate change. If you support an indigenous people's right to self-determination, if you support your local anti-fascists and people fighting police brutality; if you support demilitarisation and nuclear disarmament … it's all one planet" (Thorne, 2019: timestamp: 24:28). This pertains to the industrious and continual re-emergence of gender diverse communities, because an accessible economic environment and sustainable ecological environment are necessary precursors to survival.

This book has explored the relationship between non-binary identities, queer communities, and medical practice of all kinds. In doing so, I hope that the benefits of sociological analysis can be harnessed to pragmatically impact both systemic cultural norms and individual lives for the better.

Notes

1   It is also contended that enby was created to avoid using 'NB' due to its existent use as an abbreviation for other concepts, particularly 'non-black' and a political desire not to appropriate black community language. To illustrate, see www. anamardoll.com/2018/02/storify-why-i-use-enby-and-not-nb.html. The point has been made that while no-one 'owns' the initialism, there is cultural precedent for language originating in black communities to be marginalised in comparison to white-associated phrases. A relevant example would be how propagating NB-as-non-binary risks creating a racialised educational load, should people of colour find themselves, for example, needing to disentangle potential confusion regarding non-binary when using acronyms such as NBPOC (non-black people of colour).

2   This account was heard during a direct conversation with the professional responsible, through my membership and work with the World Professional Association for Transgender Health (WPATH).

3   Which I define here as any process of assessment where the assessor has the ability to deny the patient's autonomous access to healthcare interventions, when the patient is in receipt of knowledge and understanding of outcomes, limitations and risks in their specific context.

4   See: https://nationallgbtpartnership.org/2019/10/23/greater-manchester-trans-health-service-pilot/

5   With some exception being made for the Government Equalities Office LGBT Survey from 2018, which had more than 7,400 non-binary respondents.

References

Ackerly B and True J (2010) Back to the future: feminist theory, activism, and doing feminist research in an age of globalization. *Women's Studies International Forum* 33: 464–72

Adams N, Pearce R, Veale J, et al. (2017) Guidance and ethical considerations for undertaking transgender health research and institutional review boards adjudicating this research. *Transgender Health* 2: 165–75

Alarie M and Gaudet S (2013) 'I don't know if she is bisexual or if she just wants to get attention': analyzing the various mechanisms through which emerging adults invisibilize bisexuality. *Journal of Bisexuality* 13: 191–214

Alaszewski A (2006) *Using diaries for social research.* London/New Delhi/Thousand Oaks, CA: Sage Publications

Alfieri S and Marta E (2011) Positive attitudes toward the outgroup: adaptation and validation of the Allophilia scale. *Testing, Psychometrics, Methodology in Applied Psychology* 18: 99–116

Ashley F (2021, forthcoming) 'Trans' is my gender modality: a modest terminological proposal. In: Erickson-Schroth L (ed.) *Trans bodies, trans selves* (2nd edn). New York/Oxford: Oxford University Press

Atkinson R and Flint J (2001) Accessing hidden and hard-to-reach populations: snowball research strategies. *Social Research Update* 33: 1–4

Bailey JM (2003) *The man who would be queen: The science of gender-bending and transsexualism.* Washington DC: Joseph Henry Press

Ball JRB (1967) Transsexualism and transvestitism. *Australasian Psychiatry* 1: 188–95

Baril A and Trevenen K (2014) Exploring ableism and cisnormativity in the conceptualization of identity and sexuality 'disorders'. *Annual Review of Critical Psychology* 11: 389–416

Barker M-J and Iantaffi A (2019) *Life isn't binary.* London/Philadelphia, PA: Jessica Kingsley Publishers

Barker M (2013a) Consent is a grey area? A comparison of understandings of consent in *Fifty Shades of Grey* and on the BDSM blogosphere. *Sexualities* 16: 896–914

Barker M (2013b) Gender and BDSM revisited. Reflections on a decade of researching kink communities. *Psychology of Women Section Review* 15: 20–8

Barker M and Langdridge D (2008) II. Bisexuality: working with a silenced sexuality. *Feminism & Psychology* 18: 389–94

Baron-Cohen S (2004) *The essential difference.* London/New York: Penguin Books

Barrett J (2007) *Transsexual and other disorders of gender identity: A practical guide to management.* Oxford/New York: Radcliffe Publishing

Bauer GR, Hammond R, Travers R, et al. (2009) 'I don't think this is theoretical; this is our lives': How erasure impacts health care for transgender people. *Journal of the Association of Nurses in AIDS Care* 20: 348–61

BBC News (2019) Is it OK to take the pill every day without a break? 21 January, www.bbc.co.uk/news/health-46952694

Beauchamp T (2014) Surveillance. *Transgender Studies Quarterly* 1: 208–10

Beech N (2011) Liminality and the practices of identity reconstruction. *Human Relations* 64: 285–302

Beemyn G (2013) A presence in the past: a transgender historiography. *Journal of Women's History* 25: 113–21

Belcher H (2014) TransDocFail – the findings. 29 November. https://challengingjourneys.files.wordpress.com/2014/11/transdocfail-findings.pdf

Benjamin H (1966) *The transsexual phenomenon.* New York: The Julian Press

Benney M and Hughes EC (1956) Of sociology and the interview. *American Journal of Sociology* 62: 137–42

Benzies K and Allen M (2001) Symbolic interactionism as a theoretical perspective for multiple method research. *Journal of Advanced Nursing* 33: 541–7

Berg M (1998) Order(s) and disorder(s): of protocols and medical practices. In: Berg M and Mol A (eds) *Differences in medicine: Unraveling practices, techniques, and bodies.* London/Durham NC: Duke University Press, 226–46

Betancourt JR and Green AR (2007) Cultural competence: healthcare disparities and political issues. In: Walker PF and Barnett ED (eds) *Immigrant medicine.* Saunders Elsevier, 99–109

Bettcher TM (2014) Trapped in the wrong theory: rethinking trans oppression and resistance. *Signs* 39: 383–406

Bhat R (1999) Characteristics of private medical practice in India: a provider perspective. *Health Policy and Planning* 14: 26–37

Biernacki P and Waldorf D (1981) Snowball sampling: problems and techniques of chain referral sampling. *Sociological Methods & Research* 10: 141–63

Bilodeau B (2005) Beyond the gender binary: a case study of two transgender students at a Midwestern research university. *Journal of Gay & Lesbian Issues in Education* 3: 29–44

Bivens R (2017) The gender binary will not be deprogrammed: ten years of coding gender on Facebook. *New Media & Society* 19: 880–98

Blumer H (1969) *Symbolic interactionism: Perspective and method.* London: University of California Press

Bockting W, Robinson B, Benner A and Scheltema, K (2004) Patient satisfaction with transgender health services. *Journal of Sex & Marital Therapy* 30: 277–94

Bockting WO (2008) Psychotherapy and the real-life experience: from gender dichotomy to gender diversity. *Sexologies* 17: 211–24

Bolger N, Davis A and Rafaeli E (2003) Diary methods: capturing life as it is lived. *Annual Review of Psychology* 54: 579–616

Bolton RM (2019) Reworking testosterone as a man's hormone: non-binary people using testosterone within a binary gender system. *Somatechnics* 9: 13–31

Bornstein K (1994) *Gender outlaw: On men, women, and the rest of us.* London/New York: Routledge

Bornstein K and Bergman SB (2010) *Gender outlaws: The next generation.* Berkeley CA: Seal Press

Bouman WP, Bauer GR, Richards C, et al. (2010) World professional association for transgender health consensus statement on considerations of the role of distress (criterion d) in the DSM diagnosis of gender identity disorder. *International Journal of Transgenderism* 12: 100–6

Bradford NJ, Rider GN, Catalpa JM, et al. (2018) Creating gender: a thematic analysis of genderqueer narratives. *International Journal of Transgenderism*: 1–14

Bradshaw B and Ryan M (2012) Healthcare-related transgender bias. *The Resident's Journal* 7: 9–10

Bragg S and Buckingham D (2008) Scrapbooks as a resource in media research with young people. In: Thomson P (ed.) *Doing visual research with children and young people.* London/New York: Routledge, 114–31

Breen LJ (2007) The researcher 'in the middle': negotiating the insider/outsider dichotomy. *The Australian Community Psychologist* 19: 163–74

Bullough VL and Bullough B (1993) *Cross dressing, sex, and gender.* Philadelphia PA: University of Pennsylvania Press

Burgwal A, Gvianishvili N, Hård V, et al. (2019) Health disparities between binary and non binary trans people: a community-driven survey. *International Journal of Transgenderism*: 1–12

Butler J (1993) *Bodies that matter: On the discursive limits of 'sex'*. New York: Routledge

Califia P (2012) *Sex changes: Transgender politics*. Jersey City, NJ: Cleis Press

Callis AS (2013) The black sheep of the pink flock: labels, stigma, and bisexual identity. *Journal of Bisexuality* 13: 82–105

Campbell D (2015) 'Chronic underfunding' of social care increases burden on NHS, say GPs. *The Guardian*, 13 March. www.theguardian.com/society/2015/mar/13/chronic-underfunding-social-care-cuts-burden-nhs-gps

Carpenter M (2018) What do intersex people need from doctors? *O&G Magazine* 20(4), www.ogmagazine.org.au/20/4-20/what-do-intersex-people-need-from-doctors/

Carter J (2013) Embracing transition, or dancing in the folds of time. In: Stryker S and Aizura AZ (eds) *The transgender studies reader 2*. London/New York: Routledge, 130–43

Catalano DCJ (2015) 'Trans enough?' The pressures trans men negotiate in higher education. *TSQ: Transgender Studies Quarterly* 2: 411–30

Cauldwell D (1949) Psychopathia transsexualis. *Sexology* 16: 274–80

Cavanaugh T, Hopwood R and Lambert C (2016) Informed consent in the medical care of transgender and gender-nonconforming patients. *AMA Journal of Ethics* 18: 1147–55

Chang TK and Chung YB (2015) Transgender microaggressions: complexity of the heterogeneity of transgender identities. *Journal of LGBT Issues in Counseling* 9: 217–34

Clarke JN and James S (2003) The radicalized self: the impact on the self of the contested nature of the diagnosis of chronic fatigue syndrome. *Social Science & Medicine* 57: 1387–95

Coleman E, Bockting W, Botzer M, et al. (2012) Standards of care for the health of transsexual, transgender, and gender-nonconforming people, version 7. *International Journal of Transgenderism* 13: 165–232

Connell R (1995) *Masculinities*. London/Berkeley CA: University of California Press

Cromwell J (1999) Passing women and female-bodied men: (re)claiming FTM history. In: Whittle S and More K (eds) *Reclaiming genders: Transsexual grammars at the fin de siècle*. London/New York: Cassell, 34–61

Crossley N (2006) In the gym: motives, meaning and moral careers. *Body & Society* 12: 23–50

Currah P (2006) Gender pluralisms under the transgender umbrella. In: Currah P, Juang RM and Price Minter S (eds) *Transgender rights*. Minneapolis IN: University of Minnesota Press, 3–31

D'Augelli AR (1994) Identity development and sexual orientation: toward a model of lesbian, gay, and bisexual development. In: Trickett EJ, Watts RJ and Birman D (eds) *Human diversity: Perspectives on people in context.* San Francisco CA: Jossey-Bass, 312–33

de Vries KM (2015) Transgender people of color at the center: conceptualizing a new intersectional model. *Ethnicities* 15: 3–27

Deakin H and Wakefield K (2014) Skype interviewing: reflections of two PhD researchers. *Qualitative Research* 14: 603–16

Deutsch MB (2012) Use of the informed consent model in the provision of cross-sex hormone therapy: a survey of the practices of selected clinics. *International Journal of Transgenderism* 13: 140–6

Devlin K (2010) Patients' medical records go online without consent. *The Telegraph*, 9 March. www.telegraph.co.uk/news/health/news/7408379/Patients-medical-records-go-online-without-consent.html

Devor H (1987) Gender blending females. *American Behavioural Scientist* 31: 12–40

Devor H (1989) *Gender blending: Confronting the limits of duality.* Bloomington IN: Indiana University Press

Dewey J (1905) The realism of pragmatism. *The Journal of Philosophy, Psychology and Scientific Methods* 2: 324–7

Dewey JM (2008) Knowledge legitimacy: how trans-patient behavior supports and challenges current medical knowledge. *Qualitative Health Research* 18: 1345–55

Dewey JM (2013) Challenges of implementing collaborative models of decision making with trans-identified patients. *Health Expectations* 18: 1508–18

Dickson-Swift V, James EL, Kippen S and Liamputtong P (2009) Researching sensitive topics: qualitative research as emotion work. *Qualitative Research* 9(1): 61–79

Di Giulio G (2003) Sexuality and people living with physical or developmental disabilities: a review of key issues. *The Canadian Journal of Human Sexuality* 12: 53–68

Doan L (2013) *Disturbing practices: History, sexuality, and women's experience of modern war.* London/Chicago IL: University of Chicago Press

Drager H (2012) Transforming cyber space and the trans liberation movement: a study of transmasculine youth bloggers on Tumblr.com. [Undergraduate honors thesis] http://scholar.colorado.edu/honr_theses/318

Duggan L (2002) The new homonormativity: the sexual politics of neoliberalism. In: Russ Castronovo DDN (ed.) *Materializing democracy: Toward a revitalized cultural politics*. London/Durham NC: Duke University Press, 175–194

Earnshaw VA and Quinn DM (2012) The impact of stigma in healthcare on people living with chronic illnesses. *Journal of Health Psychology* 17: 157–68

Edelman L (2004) *No future: Queer theory and the death drive*. London/ Durham NC: Duke University Press

Ekins R and King D (1999) Towards a sociology of transgendered bodies. *The Sociological Review* 47: 580–602

Ellis SJ, Bailey L and McNeil J (2015) Trans people's experiences of mental health and gender identity services: A UK study. *Journal of Gay & Lesbian Mental Health* 19: 4–20

Ellis SJ, McNeil J and Bailey L (2014) Gender, stage of transition and situational avoidance: a UK study of trans people's experiences. *Sexual and Relationship Therapy* 29: 351–64

Emmel N (2013) *Sampling and choosing cases in qualitative research: A realist approach*. London/New Delhi/Thousand Oaks, CA: Sage Publications

England KV (1994) Getting personal: reflexivity, positionality, and feminist research. *The Professional Geographer* 46: 80–9

Epple C (1998) Coming to terms with Navajo *nádleehí*: a critique of *berdache*, 'gay', 'alternate gender' and 'two-spirit'. *American Ethnologist* 25: 267–90

Fausto-Sterling A (1993) The five sexes. *The Sciences* 33: 20–4

Fausto-Sterling A (2019) Gender/sex, sexual orientation, and identity are in the body: how did they get there? *The Journal of Sex Research*: 1–27

Feinberg L (1996) *Transgender warriors: Making history from Joan of Arc to Dennis Rodman*. Boston, MA: Beacon Press

Feldman JL and Goldberg JM (2006) Transgender primary medical care. *International Journal of Transgenderism* 9: 3–34

Fereday J and Muir-Cochrane E (2006) Demonstrating rigor using thematic analysis: a hybrid approach of inductive and deductive coding and theme development. *International Journal of Qualitative Methods* 5: 80–92

Fine C (2010) *Delusions of gender*. London: Icon Books

Fine GA (1993) The sad demise, mysterious disappearance, and glorious triumph of symbolic interactionism. *Annual Review of Sociology* 19: 61–87

Finlay L and Gough B (2003) *Reflexivity: A practical guide for researchers in health and social sciences*. Oxford: Blackwell Science

Foster GD, Wadden TA, Makris AP, et al. (2003) Primary care physicians' attitudes about obesity and its treatment. *Obesity Research* 11: 1168–77

Foucault M (1973) *The birth of the clinic.* London/New York: Routledge

Foucault M (1988) Technologies of the self. In: Martin LH, Gutman H and Hutton PH (eds) *Technologies of the self.* Amherst, MA: University of Massachusetts Press, 16–49

Fowler K, Grimstad F, New E, et al. (2018) Evaluation of ovarian pathology in transgender men and gender non-binary persons on testosterone. *Journal of Pediatric and Adolescent Gynecology* 31: 183

Fraley RC and Hudson NW (2014) Review of intensive longitudinal methods: an introduction to diary and experience sampling research. *The Journal of Social Psychology* 154: 89–91

Freeman L and López SA (2018) Sex categorization in medical contexts: a cautionary tale. *Kennedy Institute of Ethics Journal* 28: 243–80

Frohard-Dourlent H, Dobson S, Clark BA, et al. (2017) 'I would have preferred more options': accounting for non-binary youth in health research. *Nursing Inquiry* 24: e12150

Gagné P and Tewksbury R (1998) Conformity pressures and gender resistance among transgendered individuals. *Social problems* 45: 81–101

Gagné P, Tewksbury R and McGaughey D (1997) Coming out and crossing over identity formation and proclamation in a transgender community. *Gender & Society* 11: 478–508

Gagnon JH and Simon W (1974) *Sexual conduct: The social origins of human sexuality.* Chicago, IL: Aldine Press

Galupo MP, Henise SB and Mercer NL (2016) 'The labels don't work very well': transgender individuals' conceptualizations of sexual orientation and sexual identity. *International Journal of Transgenderism* 17: 93–104

Galupo MP, Pulice-Farrow L, Clements ZA, et al. (2018) 'I love you as both and I love you as neither': romantic partners' affirmations of nonbinary trans individuals. *International Journal of Transgenderism*: 1–13

Gamarel KE, Reisner SL, Laurenceau J-P, et al. (2014) Gender minority stress, mental health, and relationship quality: a dyadic investigation of transgender women and their cisgender male partners. *Journal of Family Psychology* 28: 437–47

Ganga D and Scott S (2006) Cultural 'insiders' and the issue of positionality in qualitative migration research: moving 'across' and moving 'along' researcher-participant divides. *Forum Qualitative Sozialforschung/Forum: Qualitative Social Research* 7: 1–12

Garfinkel H (2006) Passing and the managed achievement of sex status in an 'intersexed' person. In: Susan Stryker and Whittle S (eds) *The transgender studies reader*. New York: Routledge, 58–93

Garrison S (2018) On the limits of 'trans enough': authenticating trans identity narratives. *Gender & Society* 32: 613–37

Gill R and Elias AS (2014) 'Awaken your incredible': love your body discourses and postfeminist contradictions. *International Journal of Media & Cultural Politics* 10: 179–88

Giordano J, O'Reilly M, Taylor H, et al. (2007) Confidentiality and autonomy: the challenge(s) of offering research participants a choice of disclosing their identity. *Qualitative Health Research* 17: 264–75

Glaser BG and Strauss AL (1999) *The discovery of grounded theory: Strategies for qualitative research*. Piscataway, NJ: Transaction Publishers

Goffman E (1959) *The presentation of self in everyday life*. New York: Anchor Books

Goffman E (1997) Selections from stigma. In: Davis LJ (ed.) *The disability studies reader*. London/New York: Routledge, 203–15

Government Equalities Office (2018) National LGBT Survey: Research report. London: Department for Education

Grady D, Gebretsadik T, Kerlikowske K, et al. (1995) Hormone replacement therapy and endometrial cancer risk: a meta-analysis. *Obstetrics & Gynecology* 85: 304–13

Gran J, Bhatia V, Davies A, et al. (2019) Non-binary population size in a large national UK gender identity clinic. *EPATH 2019*. Rome

Grant JM, Mottet L, Tanis JE, et al. (2011) *Injustice at every turn: A report of the National Transgender Discrimination Survey*. www.transequality. org/sites/default/files/docs/resources/NTDS_Report.pdf

Griffith AI (1998) Insider/outsider: epistemological privilege and mothering work. *Human Studies* 21: 361–76

Grimstad F, Fowler K, New E, et al. (2018) Evaluation of uterine pathology in transgender men and gender nonbinary persons on testosterone. *Journal of Pediatric and Adolescent Gynecology* 31: 217

Guest G, Bunce A and Johnson L (2006) How many interviews are enough? An experiment with data saturation and variability. *Field Methods* 18: 59–82

Haas AP, Rodgers PL and Herman JL (2014) *Suicide attempts among transgender and gender non-conforming adults*. https://williamsinstitute. law.ucla.edu/wp-content/uploads/AFSP-Williams-Suicide-Report-Final.pdf

Hagen DB and Galupo MP (2014) Trans* individuals' experiences of gendered language with health care providers: recommendations for practitioners. *International Journal of Transgenderism* 15: 16–34

Halberstam J (1998) *Female masculinity*. London/Durham NC: Duke University Press

Halberstam J (2005) *In a queer time and place: Transgender bodies, subcultural lives*. London/New York: New York University Press

Hale J (1996) Are lesbians women? *Hypatia* 11: 94–121

Hall MA and Schneider CE (2008) Patients as consumers: courts, contracts, and the new medical marketplace. *Michigan Law Review* 106: 643–89

Hamati-Ataya I (2014) Transcending objectivism, subjectivism, and the knowledge in-between: the subject in/of 'strong reflexivity'. *Review of International Studies* 40: 153–75

Haraway D (1988) Situated knowledges: the science question in feminism and the privilege of partial perspective. *Feminist Studies* 14: 575–99

Harding S (1983) Why has the sex/gender system become visible only now? In: Harding S and Hintikka MB (eds) *Discovering reality: Feminist perspectives on epistemology, metaphysics, methodology, and philosophy of science*. Dordrecht: Springer, 311–24

Harrison J, Grant J and Herman JL (2012) A gender not listed here: genderqueers, gender rebels, and otherwise in the National Transgender Discrimination Survey. *LGBTQ Public Policy Journal at the Harvard Kennedy School* 2: 13–24

Hausman BL (1995) *Changing sex: Transsexualism, technology, and the idea of gender*. London/Durham NC: Duke University Press

Hegarty P, Ansara YG and Barker M-J (2018) Nonbinary gender identities. In: Dess NK, Marecek J and Bell LC (eds) *Gender, sex, and sexualities: Psychological perspectives*. New York: Oxford University Press, 53–76

Heilman ME (1995) Sex stereotypes and their effects in the workplace: what we know and what we don't know. *Journal of Social Behavior and Personality* 10: 3–26

Hendricks ML and Testa RJ (2012) A conceptual framework for clinical work with transgender and gender nonconforming clients: an adaptation of the minority stress model. *Professional Psychology-Research and Practice* 43: 460–7

Herdt GH (1993) *Third sex, third gender: Beyond sexual dimorphism in culture and history*. New York: Zone Books

Herman JL (2013) Gendered restrooms and minority stress: the public regulation of gender and its impact on transgender people's lives. *Journal of Public Management & Social Policy* 19: 65–80

Hill DA, Weiss NS, Beresford SA, et al. (2000) Continuous combined hormone replacement therapy and risk of endometrial cancer. *American Journal of Obstetrics and Gynecology* 183: 1456–61

Hines S (2006) What's the difference? Bringing particularity to queer studies of transgender. *Journal of Gender Studies* 15: 49–66

Hines S (2007a) *Transforming gender: Transgender practices of identity, intimacy and care*. London: Policy Press

Hines S (2007b) Transgendering care: practices of care within transgender communities. *Critical Social Policy* 27: 462–86

Hines S (2010) Queerly situated? Exploring negotiations of trans queer subjectivities at work and within community spaces in the UK. *Gender, Place and Culture* 17: 597–613

Hines S (2013) *Gender diversity, recognition and citizenship: Towards a politics of difference*. London: Palgrave Macmillan

Hines S and Sanger T (2010) *Transgender identities: towards a social analysis of gender diversity*. London/New York: Routledge

Hird MJ (2000) Gender's nature: intersexuality, transsexualism and the 'sex'/'gender' binary. *Feminist Theory* 1: 347–64

Hird MJ (2002) For a sociology of transsexualism. *Sociology* 36: 577–95

Hirschfeld M (1910) *Die Transvestiten: eine Untersuchung über den erotischen Verkleidungstrieb: mit umfangreichen casuistischen und historischen Material*. Berlin: A. Pulvermacher

Hirschfeld M (1923) Die intersexuelle konstitution. *Jahrbuch für sexuelle Zwischenstufen* 23: 3–27

Hirschkorn KA (2006) Exclusive versus everyday forms of professional knowledge: legitimacy claims in conventional and alternative medicine. *Sociology of Health & Illness* 28: 533–57

Hochschild AR (2012) *The managed heart: Commercialization of human feeling*. Berkeley, CA: University of California Press

Holliday R (2000) We've been framed: visualising methodology. *The Sociological Review* 48: 503–21

Horak L (2014) Trans on YouTube: intimacy, visibility, temporality. *Transgender Studies Quarterly* 1: 572–85

Horvath KJ, Beadnell B and Bowen AM (2007) A daily web diary of the sexual experiences of men who have sex with men: comparisons with a retrospective recall survey. *AIDS and Behavior* 11: 537–48

House of Commons Women and Equalities Committee (2016) *Transgender equality: First report of session 2015–16*. London: The Stationery Office

Hupf R (2015) Allyship to the intersex community on cosmetic, non-consensual genital normalizing surgery. *William & Mary Journal of Race, Gender, and Social Justice* 22: 73–104

Huxter W (2016) Improving awareness and understanding of transgender issues. [Blog] 9 September, NHS England. www.england. nhs.uk/2016/09/will-huxter-14/

Hyers LL, Swim JK and Mallett RK (2006) Personal is political: using daily diaries to examine everyday prejudice-related experiences. In: Hesse-Biber SN and Leavy P (eds) *Emergent methods in social research.* London/ New Delhi/Thousand Oaks, CA: Sage Publications, 313–35

Iida M, Shrout PE, Laurenceau J-P, et al. (2012) Using diary methods in psychological research. In: Cooper H, Camic PM, Long DL, et al. (eds) *APA handbook of research methods in psychology, Vol 1: Foundations, planning, measures, and psychometrics.* Washington, DC: American Psychological Association, 277–305

Ingraham C (1994) The heterosexual imaginary: feminist sociology and theories of gender. *Sociological Theory* 12: 203–19

Irvine A, Drew P and Sainsbury R (2013) 'Am I not answering your questions properly?' Clarification, adequacy and responsiveness in semi-structured telephone and face-to-face interviews. *Qualitative Research* 13: 87–106

Jackson S and Scott S (2010) Rehabilitating interactionism for a feminist sociology of sexuality. *Sociology* 44: 811–26

Jacobs SE (1968) Berdache: a brief review of the literature. *Colorado Anthropologist* 1: 25–40

Jeffreys S (2014) *Gender hurts: A feminist analysis of the politics of transgenderism.* London/New York: Routledge

Johnson AH (2016) Transnormativity: a new concept and its validation through documentary film about transgender men. *Sociological Inquiry* 86: 465–91

Julienne, A (2018) Revisiting the life of trailblazing queer heroine Annemarie Schwarzenbach. *Dazed,* 2 November. www.dazeddigital. com/art-photography/article/42063/1/queer-icon-annemarie-schwarzenbach-photographer-writer-givenchy-ss19

Kanuha VK (2000) 'Being' native versus 'going native': conducting social work research as an insider. *Social Work* 45: 439–47

Kattari SK, Walls NE and Speer SR (2017) Differences in experiences of discrimination in accessing social services among transgender/ gender nonconforming individuals by (dis)ability. *Journal of Social Work in Disability & Rehabilitation* 16: 116–40

Keatley J (2015) What it was like to transition 50 years ago. *Daily Beast,* 11 July. www.thedailybeast.com/articles/2015/07/11/what-it-was-like-to-transition-50-years-ago.html

Kennedy N (2013) Cultural cisgenderism: consequences of the imperceptible. *Psychology of Women Section Review* 15: 3–11

Kennedy N (2019) Becoming: discourses of trans emergence, epiphanies and oppositions. In: Pearce R, Moon I and Gupta KS, Steinberg DL (eds) *The emergence of trans: Cultures, politics and everyday lives.* London: Routledge, 46–59

Kennedy P (2008) *The first man-made man: The story of two sex changes, one love affair, and a twentieth-century medical revolution.* New York: Bloomsbury Publishing

Kerr EA, Hays RD, Mitchinson A, et al. (1999) The influence of gatekeeping and utilization review on patient satisfaction. *Journal of General Internal Medicine* 14: 287–96

Kessler SJ and McKenna W (1978) *Gender: An ethnomethodological approach*, Chicago, IL: University of Chicago Press

King J (2016) If you're transgender, there's no such thing as a routine doctor's visit. *Mic*, 29 June. https://mic.com/articles/147317/if-you-re-transgender-there-s-no-such-thing-as-a-routine-doctor-s-visit#. V4erI3zck

Kinne S, Patrick DL and Doyle DL (2004) Prevalence of secondary conditions among people with disabilities. *American Journal of Public Health* 94: 443–5

Kobayashi A (2001) Negotiating the personal and the political in critical qualitative research. In: Limb M and Dwyer C (eds) *Qualitative methodologies for geographers: Issues and debates.* London/New York: Arnold Publishers, 55–70

Kong TS, Mahoney D and Plummer K (2001) Queering the interview. In: Gubrium JF and Holstein JA (eds) *Handbook of interview research.* London/New Delhi/Thousand Oaks, CA: Sage Publications, 91–110

Kosenko K, Rintamaki L, Raney S, et al. (2013) Transgender patient perceptions of stigma in health care contexts. *Medical Care* 51: 819–22

Larson EB and Yao X (2005) Clinical empathy as emotional labor in the patient-physician relationship. *JAMA* 293: 1100–6

LaSala MC (2003) When interviewing 'family' maximizing the insider advantage in the qualitative study of lesbians and gay men. *Journal of Gay & Lesbian Social Services* 15: 15–30

Lee RM (1993) *Researching sensitive topics.* London: Sage Publications

Leeds-Hurwitz W (2006) Social theories: social constructionism and symbolic interactionism. In: Braithwaite DO (ed.) *Engaging theories in family communication: Multiple perspectives.* London/New Delhi/Thousand Oaks, CA: Sage Publications, 229–42

Leeds and York Partnership NHS Foundation Trust (2020) Gender identity service. www.leedsandyorkpft.nhs.uk/our-services/services-list/gender-identity-service/

Levine SB (2009) Real-life test experience: recommendations for revisions to the standards of care of the World Professional Association for Transgender Health. *International Journal of Transgenderism* 11: 186–93

Levitt HM and Ippolito MR (2014) Being transgender: the experience of transgender identity development. *Journal of Homosexuality* 61: 1727–58

Lewis CL, Wickstrom GC, Kolar MM, et al. (2000) Patient preferences for care by general internists and specialists in the ambulatory setting. *Journal of General Internal Medicine* 15: 75–83

Lewis JD and Smith RL (1980) *American sociology and pragmatism: Mead, Chicago sociology, and symbolic interaction.* London/Chicago, IL: University of Chicago Press

Lin JT and Mathew P (2005) Cancer pain management in prisons: a survey of primary care practitioners and inmates. *Journal of Pain and Symptom Management* 29: 466–73

Lingiardi V and McWilliams N (2017) *Psychodynamic diagnostic manual: PDM-2.* New York: Guilford Publications

Little M, Jordens CF, Paul K, et al. (1998) Liminality: a major category of the experience of cancer illness. *Social Science & Medicine* 47: 1485–94

Lorber J (1975) Good patients and problem patients: conformity and deviance in a general hospital. *Journal of Health and Social Behavior* 16: 213–25

Losty M and O'Connor J (2018) Falling outside of the 'nice little binary box': a psychoanalytic exploration of the non-binary gender identity. *Psychoanalytic Psychotherapy* 32: 40–60

Loudon I (2008) The principle of referral: the gatekeeping role of the GP. *British Journal of General Practice* 58: 128–30

Love H (2014) Queer. *Transgender Studies Quarterly* 1: 172–6

Lurie NO (1953) Winnebago berdache. *American Anthropologist* 55: 708–12

Lyons K (2016) Gender identity clinic services under strain as referral rates soar. *The Guardian*, 10 July. www.theguardian.com/society/2016/jul/10/transgender-clinic-waiting-times-patient-numbers-soar-gender-identity-services

Malinowski B (1927) *Sex and repression in savage society.* London/New York: Kegan Paul, Trench, Trubner & Co. Ltd

Marciano A (2014) Living the virtureal: negotiating transgender identity in cyberspace. *Journal of Computer-Mediated Communication* 19: 824–38

Martínez-Iñigo D, Totterdell P, Alcover CM, et al. (2007) Emotional labour and emotional exhaustion: interpersonal and intrapersonal mechanisms. *Work & Stress* 21: 30–47

Mason M (2010) Sample size and saturation in PhD studies using qualitative interviews. *Forum: Qualitative Social Research/Sozialforschung* 11(3).

Matsuno E and Budge SL (2017) Non-binary/genderqueer identities: a critical review of the literature. *Current Sexual Health Reports* 9: 116–20

Mauthner NS and Doucet A (2003) Reflexive accounts and accounts of reflexivity in qualitative data analysis. *Sociology* 37: 413–31

McCormack M (2013) *The declining significance of homophobia*. Oxford/ New York: Oxford University Press

McLeod ME (2003) The caring physician: a journey in self-exploration and self-care. *The American Journal of Gastroenterology* 98: 2135–8

McNeil J, Bailey L, Ellis S, Morton J and Regan M (2012) *Trans mental health study 2012*. Edinburgh: Scottish Transgender Alliance

Mead GH (1934) *Mind, self, and society: From the standpoint of a social behaviorist*. London/Chicago IL: University of Chicago Press

Mol A (1999) Ontological politics. A word and some questions. *The Sociological Review* 47: 74–89

Monro S (2003) Transgender politics in the UK. *Critical Social Policy* 23: 433–52

Monro S (2005a) *Gender politics: Citizenship, activism and sexual diversity.* London: Pluto Press

Monro S (2005b) Beyond male and female: poststructuralism and the spectrum of gender. *International Journal of Transgenderism* 8: 3–22

Monro S (2007) Transmuting gender binaries: the theoretical challenge. *Sociological Research Online* 12: 1–15

Monro S (2015) *Bisexuality: Identities, politics, and theories.* London: Palgrave Macmillan

Monro S (2019) Non-binary and genderqueer: an overview of the field. *International Journal of Transgenderism* 2–3: 126–31

Monro S and Richardson D (2014) Citizenship, gender and sexuality. In: Heijden H-Avd (ed.) *Handbook of political citizenship and social movements*. Cheltenham/Northampton, MA: Edward Elgar Publishing Ltd, 60–86

Monro S and Warren L (2004) Transgendering citizenship. *Sexualities* 7: 345–62

Montgomery D (1994) The Charing Cross Gender Identity Unit. [Report of presentation] GENDYS '94, The Third International Gender Dysphoria Conference. Manchester, England. www.gender. org.uk/conf/1994/index.htm#montgomery

Moore S, Gridley H, Taylor K, et al. (2000) Women's views about intimate examinations and sexually inappropriate practices by their general practitioners. *Psychology and Health* 15: 71–84

Motmans J, Nieder TO and Bouman WP (2019) Transforming the paradigm of nonbinary transgender health: a field in transition. *International Journal of Transgenderism*: 1–8

Muñoz JE (2009) *Cruising utopia: The then and there of queer futurity.* New York: New York University Press

Murad MH, Elamin MB, Garcia MZ, et al. (2010) Hormonal therapy and sex reassignment: a systematic review and meta-analysis of quality of life and psychosocial outcomes. *Clinical Endocrinology* 72: 214–31

Mutch C, Marlowe J, Robinson M, et al. (2013) Gender and sexual minorities: intersecting inequalities and health. *Ethnicity and Inequalities in Health and Social Care* 6: 91–6

Namaste V (2000) *Invisible lives: The erasure of transsexual and transgendered people.* London/Chicago IL: University of Chicago Press

Nanda S (1990) *Neither man nor woman: The Hijras of India.* Belmont, CA: Wadsworth Publishing Company

Neal OR (1995) The limits of legal discourse: learning from the civil rights movement in the quest for gay and lesbian civil rights. *New York Law School Law Review* 40: 679–718

Neff K (2003) Self-compassion: an alternative conceptualization of a healthy attitude toward oneself. *Self and Identity* 2: 85–101

Nestle J, Howell C and Wilchins RA (2002) *Genderqueer: Voices from beyond the sexual binary.* Los Angeles/New York: Alyson Publications

Newman J and Vidler E (2006) Discriminating customers, responsible patients, empowered users: consumerism and the modernisation of health care. *Journal of Social Policy* 35: 193–209

NHS (2016) Types: Hormone replacement therapy (HRT). www.nhs. uk/conditions/hormone-replacement-therapy-hrt/types/

NHS England (2013) Interim NHS England gender dysphoria protocol and service guideline 2013/14. www.gires.org.uk/wp-content/ uploads/2017/03/int-gend-proto.pdf

NHS England (2016) NHS England response to the specific duties of the Equality Act. www.england.nhs.uk/wp-content/uploads/2016/02/ nhse-specific-duties-equality-act.pdf

NHS England (2018) Service specifications for gender identity services for adults (non-surgical interventions). www.engage.england.nhs.uk/survey/gender-identity-services-for-adults/user_uploads/specialised-gender-dysphoria-service-specifications.pdf

Nicholas L (2018) Queer ethics and fostering positive mindsets toward non-binary gender, genderqueer, and gender ambiguity. *International Journal of Transgenderism*: 1–12

Nicholson L and Seidman S (1995) *Social postmodernism: Beyond identity politics*. Cambridge: Cambridge University Press

Niemietz K (2016) Rebuttal: 'The NHS is wonderful, just underfunded'. [Blog] Institute of Economic Affairs, 13 January. https://iea.org.uk/blog/rebuttal-the-nhs-is-wonderful-just-underfunded

Nirta C (2017) *Marginal bodies, trans utopias*. London: Routledge

Nordmarken S (2014) Becoming ever more monstrous feeling transgender in-betweenness. *Qualitative Inquiry* 20: 37–50

Nottinghamshire Healthcare NHS Foundation Trust (2016) Frequently asked questions. Nottingham Centre for Transgender Health. www.nottinghamshirehealthcare.nhs.uk/gender-faqs

Oakley A (1981) Interviewing women: a contradiction in terms. In: Roberts H (ed.) *Doing feminist research*. London/New York: Routledge, 30–61

Obedin-Maliver J, Goldsmith ES, Stewart L, et al. (2011) Lesbian, gay, bisexual, and transgender-related content in undergraduate medical education. *JAMA* 306: 971–7

Ochoa M (2008) Perverse citizenship: divas, marginality, and participation in 'loca-lization'. *WSQ: Women's Studies Quarterly* 36: 146–69

Parsons T (1951) *The social system*. New York: The Free Press

Pearce R (2012) Inadvertent praxis: what can 'genderfork' tell us about trans feminism? *MP: An Online Feminist Journal* 3: 87–129

Pearce R (2018) *Understanding trans health: Discourse, power and possibility*. Bristol: Policy Press

Pearce R (2019) Trans temporalities and non-linear ageing. In: King A, Almack K, Suen Y-T, et al. (eds) *Older lesbian, gay, bisexual and trans people: Minding the knowledge gaps*. London: Routledge

Pearce R and Lohman K (2019) De/constructing DIY identities in a trans music scene. *Sexualities* 22: 97–113

Pellegrino ED (1986) Rationing health care: the ethics of medical gatekeeping. *Journal of Contemporary Health, Law & Policy* 2: 23–46

Pencheon D (1998) Managing demand: matching demand and supply fairly and efficiently. *British Medical Journal* 316: 1665–7

Person E and Ovesey L (1974a) The transsexual syndrome in males: I. Primary transsexualism. *American Journal of Psychotherapy* 28: 4–20

Person E and Ovesey L (1974b) The transsexual syndrome in males: II. Secondary transsexualism. *American Journal of Psychotherapy* 28: 174–93

Peter E and Watt-Watson J (2002) Unrelieved pain: an ethical and epistemological analysis of distrust in patients. *The Canadian Journal of Nursing Research* 34: 65–80

PinkNews (2009) Trans groups to campaign over 'draconian' gender clinic rules. 5 May. www.pinknews.co.uk/2009/05/05/trans-groups-to-campaign-over-draconian-gender-clinic-rules/

Plemons E (2019) Reconceiving the body: a surgical genealogy of trans-therapeutics. In: Pearce R, Moon I and Gupta KS, Steinberg DL (eds) *The emergence of trans: Cultures, politics and everyday lives*. London: Routledge, 34–44

Plummer K (1995) *Telling sexual stories: Power, change, and social worlds*. London/New York: Routledge

Plummer K (2003) Queers, bodies and postmodern sexualities: a note on revisiting the 'sexual' in symbolic interactionism. *Qualitative Sociology* 26: 515–30

Poteat T, German D and Kerrigan D (2013) Managing uncertainty: a grounded theory of stigma in transgender health care encounters. *Social Science & Medicine* 84: 22–9

Prescott N (2019) Transgender people wait years for help in clinic system at 'breaking point'. *The Meteor*, 7 May. www.themeteor.org/2019/05/07/transgender-people-wait-years-for-help-in-a-gender-clinic-system-at-breaking-point/

Prince V (2005) Sex vs. gender. *International Journal of Transgenderism* 8: 29–32

Pulice-Farrow L, McNary SB and Galupo MP (2019) 'Bigender is just a Tumblr thing': microaggressions in the romantic relationships of gender non-conforming and agender transgender individuals. *Sexual and Relationship Therapy*: 1–20

Pym H (2016) Is the NHS underdoctored, underfunded and overstretched? BBC News, 3 May. www.bbc.co.uk/news/health-36198952

Rajunov M and Duane AS (2019) *Nonbinary: Memoirs of gender and identity*. Chichester/New York: Columbia University Press

Raymond JG (1979) *The transsexual empire: The making of the she-male*. Boston: Beacon Press

Richards C, Arcelus J, Barrett J, et al. (2015) Trans is not a disorder – but should still receive funding. *Sexual and Relationship Therapy* 30: 309–13

Richards C, Barker M, Lenihan P, et al. (2014) Who watches the watchmen? A critical perspective on the theorization of trans people and clinicians. *Feminism & Psychology* 24: 248–58

Richards C, Bouman WP and Barker M-J (2017) *Genderqueer and non-binary genders*. London: Palgrave Macmillan

Richards C, Bouman WP, Seal L, et al. (2016) Non-binary or genderqueer genders. *International Review of Psychiatry* 28: 95–102

Richards C and Doyle J (2018) Detransition rate in a large national UK gender identity clinic. WPATH 2018 Biannual Conference, 3–6 November, Buenos Aires, Argentina

Richardson D (1998) Sexuality and citizenship. *Sociology* 32: 83–100

Richardson D (2005) Desiring sameness? The rise of a neoliberal politics of normalisation. *Antipode* 37: 515–35

Richardson D (2007) Patterned fluidities: (re)Imagining the relationship between gender and sexuality. *Sociology* 41: 457–74

Rimes KA, Goodship N, Ussher G, et al. (2019) Non-binary and binary transgender youth: comparison of mental health, self-harm, suicidality, substance use and victimization experiences. *International Journal of Transgenderism* 20: 230–40

Rinken S (2000) The 'diagnosis of the self'. In: *The AIDS crisis and the modern self*. Dordrecht: Springer, 56–92

Ritzer G (2008) *Sociological theory*. New York: McGraw Hill

Roen K (2002) 'Either/or' and 'both/neither': discursive tensions in transgender politics. *Signs* 27: 501–22

Rogers WA (2002) Is there a moral duty for doctors to trust patients? *Journal of Medical Ethics* 28: 77–80

Rollins J and Hirsch HN (2003) Sexual identities and political engagements: a queer survey. *Social Politics* 10: 290–313

Roughgarden J (2013) *Evolution's rainbow: Diversity, gender, and sexuality in nature and people*. London/Berkeley, CA: University of California Press

Roxie M (2011) The non-binary vs genderqueer quandary. [Blog] *Genderqueer and Non-Binary Identities*, 18 October. https://genderqueerid.com/post/11617933299/the-non-binary-vs-genderqueer-quandary

Sandahl C (2003) Queering the crip or cripping the queer? Intersections of queer and crip identities in solo autobiographical performance. *GLQ: A Journal of Lesbian and Gay Studies* 9: 25–56

Sandelowski M (1995) Qualitative analysis: what it is and how to begin. *Research in Nursing & Health* 18: 371–5

Sanger T (2008) Trans governmentality: the production and regulation of gendered subjectivities. *Journal of Gender Studies* 17: 41–53

Saxey E (2008) *Homoplot: The coming-out story and gay, lesbian and bisexual identity*. New York: Peter Lang Publishing

Schilt K and Waszkiewicz E (2006) I feel so much more in my body: challenging the significance of the penis in transsexual men's bodies. [Presentation] Annual Meeting of the American Sociological Association, 13 August, Montreal, Canada

Schilt K and Westbrook L (2009) Doing gender, doing heteronormativity 'gender normals,' transgender people, and the social maintenance of heterosexuality. *Gender & Society* 23: 440–64

Schmitt S (2013) Checking our privilege, working together: notes on virtual trans★ communities, truscum blogs, and the politics of transgender health care. *The Feminist Wire*, 29 July. http:// thefeministwire.com/2013/07/checking-our-privilege-working-together-notes-on-virtual-trans-communities-truscum-blogs-and-the-politics-of-transgender-health-care/

Schroder KE, Carey MP and Vanable PA (2003) Methodological challenges in research on sexual risk behavior: II. Accuracy of self-reports. *Annals of Behavioral Medicine* 26: 104–23

Schuman H (1982) Artifacts are in the mind of the beholder. *The American Sociologist* 17(1): 21–8

Seidman S (ed.) (1996) *Queer theory sociology*. Oxford: Blackwell

Serano J (2007) *Whipping girl: A transsexual woman on sexism and the scapegoating of femininity*. Berkeley, CA: Seal Press

Shugar DR (1999) To(o) queer or not? Queer theory, lesbian community, and the functions of sexual identities. *Journal of Lesbian Studies* 3: 11–20

Shuster SM (2019) Performing informed consent in transgender medicine. *Social Science & Medicine* 226: 190–7

Singer TB (2006) From the medical gaze to sublime mutations: the ethics of (re)viewing non-normative body images. In: Stryker S and Whittle S (eds) *The transgender studies reader*. London/New York: Routledge, 601–20

Singh AA and Burnes TR (2010) Shifting the counselor role from gatekeeping to advocacy: ten strategies for using the competencies for counseling with transgender clients for individual and social change. *Journal of LGBT Issues in Counseling* 4: 241–55

Singh AA, Hays DG and Watson LS (2011) Strength in the face of adversity: resilience strategies of transgender individuals. *Journal of Counseling & Development* 89: 20–7

Slater J and Liddiard K (2018) Why disability studies scholars must challenge transmisogyny and transphobia. *Canadian Journal of Disability Studies* 7: 83–93

Spade D (2003) Resisting medicine, re/modelling gender. *Berkeley Women's Law Journal* 18: 15–35

Spade D (2004) Fighting to win. In: Sycamore MB (ed.) *That's revolting! Queer strategies for resisting assimilation.* Berkeley, CA: Soft Skull, 47–53

Spade D (2006) Mutilating gender. In: Stryker S and Whittle S (eds) *The transgender studies reader.* London/New York: Routledge, 315–32

Spivak GC (1985) Three women's texts and a critique of imperialism. *Critical Inquiry* 12: 243–61

Steedman C (1987) *Landscape for a good woman: A story of two lives.* New Brunswick, NJ: Rutgers University Press

Steinmetz K (2014) The transgender tipping point. *Time*, 29 May. http://time.com/135480/transgender-tipping-point/

Stevens S (2014) The 'patronising' gene. [Blog] *HuffPost*, 7 August. www.huffingtonpost.co.uk/simon-stevens/patronising-disabled-people_b_5562886.html

Stewart DC and Sullivan TJ (1982) Illness behavior and the sick role in chronic disease: the case of multiple sclerosis. *Social Science & Medicine* 16: 1397–404

Stoller RJ (1964) A contribution to the study of gender identity. *The International Journal of Psychoanalysis* 45: 220–6

Stoltenberg J (2005) *Refusing to be a man: Essays on social justice.* New York: Routledge

Stone S (2006) The empire strikes back: a posttranssexual manifesto. In: Stryker S and Whittle S (eds) *The transgender studies reader.* London/New York: Routledge, 221–235

Stryker S (1994) My words to Victor Frankenstein above the village of Chamounix: performing transgender rage. *GLQ* 1: 237–54

Stryker S (2008a) *Transgender history.* Berkeley, CA: Seal Press

Stryker S (2008b) Transgender history, homonormativity, and disciplinarity. *Radical History Review*: 145–57

Stryker S and Whittle S (2006) *The transgender studies reader.* London/New York: Routledge

Sullivan JR (2012) Skype: an appropriate method of data collection for qualitative interviews. *The Hilltop Review* 6: 54–60

Tagonist A (2009) Fuck you and fuck your fucking thesis: why I will not participate in trans studies. [Blog] *LiveJournal*, 10 December. https://tagonist.livejournal.com/199563.html

Tauchert A (2002) Fuzzy gender: between female-embodiment and intersex. *Journal of Gender Studies* 11: 29–38

Taylor D and Bury M (2007) Chronic illness, expert patients and care transition. *Sociology of Health & Illness* 29: 27–45

Taylor J, Zalewska A, Gates JJ, et al. (2018) An exploration of the lived experiences of non-binary individuals who have presented at a gender identity clinic in the United Kingdom. *International Journal of Transgenderism*: 1–10

Taylor V and Whittier N (1999) Collective identity in social movement communities: lesbian feminist mobilization. In: Freeman J and Johnson V (eds) *Waves of protest: Social movements since the sixties*. New York/Oxford: Rowman & Littlefield, 169–94

Taywaditep KJ (2002) Marginalization among the marginalized: gay men's anti-effeminacy attitudes. *Journal of Homosexuality* 42: 1–28

Tedlock B (1991) From participant observation to the observation of participation: the emergence of narrative ethnography. *Journal of Anthropological Research* 47: 69–94

Thomson R and Holland J (2003) Hindsight, foresight and insight: the challenges of longitudinal qualitative research. *International Journal of Social Research Methodology* 6: 233–44

Thorne O (2019) Climate grief | PhilosophyTube. [Video] 22 August. www.youtube.com/watch?v=CqCx9xU_-Fw

Thorne SE, Nyhlin KT and Paterson BL (2000) Attitudes toward patient expertise in chronic illness. *International Journal of Nursing Studies* 37: 303–311

Throsby K (2016) Unlikely becomings: passion, swimming and learning to love the sea. In: Brown M and Humberstone B (eds) *Seascapes: Shaped by the sea*. London/New York: Routledge, 155–72

Tishelman C and Sachs L (1998) The diagnostic process and the boundaries of normality. *Qualitative Health Research* 8: 48–60

Titman N (2014) How many people in the United Kingdom are nonbinary? [Blog] Practical Androgyny, 16 December. http://practicalandrogyny.com/2014/12/16/how-many-people-in-the-uk-are-nonbinary/

Tompkins A (2014) Asterisk. *Transgender Studies Quarterly* 1(1–2): 26–7

Trumbach R (1993) London's sapphists: from three sexes to four genders in the making of modern culture. In: Herdt G (ed.) *Third sex, third gender: Beyond sexual dimorphism in culture and history*. New York: Zone Books, 111–36

Tuckett AG (2005) Applying thematic analysis theory to practice: a researcher's experience. *Contemporary Nurse* 19: 75–87

Turner BS (1995) *Medical power and social knowledge*. London/New Delhi/Thousand Oaks, CA: Sage Publications

Turner DW (2010) Qualitative interview design: a practical guide for novice investigators. *The Qualitative Report* 15: 754–60

UK Trans Info (2016) Current waiting times & patient population for gender identity clinics in the UK. 25 January. https://oasisnorfolk. files.wordpress.com/2016/04/patientpopulation-oct15.pdf

Ulrichs KH ([1864] 1994) *The riddle of man-manly love: The pioneering work on male homosexuality.* New York: Prometheus Books

Usdan SL, Schumacher JE and Bernhardt JM (2004) Impaired driving behaviors among college students: a comparison of web-based daily assessment and retrospective timeline followback. *Journal of Alcohol and Drug Education* 48: 38–50

Valentine V (2016a) Non-binary people's experiences of using UK gender identity clinics. Scottish Trans Equality Network. www. scottishtrans.org/wp-content/uploads/2016/11/Non-binary-GIC-mini-report.pdf

Valentine V (2016b) Including non-binary people: guidance for service providers and employers. Scottish Trans Equality Network. www.scottishtrans.org/wp-content/uploads/2016/11/Non-binary-guidance.pdf

Valentine V (2016c) Non-binary people's experiences in the UK. Scottish Trans Equality Network. www.scottishtrans.org/wp-content/uploads/2016/11/Non-binary-report.pdf

Van Gennep A (1960) *The rites of passage.* London/Chicago IL: University of Chicago Press

Vidal-Ortiz S (2008) Transgender and transsexual studies: sociology's influence and future steps. *Sociology Compass* 2: 433–50

Vincent B (2019) Breaking down barriers and binaries in trans healthcare: the validation of non-binary people. *International Journal of Transgenderism*: 1–7

Vincent B (2018a) *Transgender health: A practitioner's guide to binary and non-binary trans patient care.* London/Philadelphia, PA: Jessica Kingsley Publishers

Vincent B (2018b) Studying trans: recommendations for ethical recruitment and collaboration with transgender participants in academic research. *Psychology & Sexuality* 9: 102–16

Vincent B and Manzano A (2017) History and cultural diversity. In: Richards C, Bouman WP and Barker M-J (eds) *Genderqueer and non-binary genders.* London: Palgrave Macmillan

Ware NC (1992) Suffering and the social construction of illness: the delegitimation of illness experience in chronic fatigue syndrome. *Medical Anthropology Quarterly* 6: 347–61

Warner LS (2013) Research as activism. In: Boyer PG and Davis DJ (eds) *Social justice issues and racism in the college classroom: Perspectives from different voices.* Bingley: Emerald Group Publishing, 133–50

Wasserfall R (1993) Reflexivity, feminism and difference. *Qualitative Sociology* 16: 23–41

Whisman V (1996) *Queer by choice: Lesbians, gay men, and the politics of identity*. New York/Abingdon: Routledge

Whitley CT (2013) Trans-kin undoing and redoing gender: negotiating relational identity among friends and family of transgender persons. *Sociological Perspectives* 56: 597–621

Whitney C (2006) Intersections in identity: identity development among queer women with disabilities. *Sexuality and Disability* 24: 39–52

WHO (World Health Organization) (2016) *The ICD-10 classification of mental and behavioural disorders: Clinical descriptions and diagnostic guidelines*. https://icd.who.int/browse10/2016/en#/F64.0

Wilchins R (1995) A note from your editrix. *In Your Face: Political Activism Against Gender Oppression* Spring: 4

Wilchins R (2002) It's your gender, stupid! In: Nestle J, Howell C and Wilchins RA (eds) *Genderqueer: Voices from beyond the sexual binary*. Los Angeles/New York: Alyson Publications, 23–32

Williams JP (2008) Symbolic interactionism. In: Given LM (ed.) *The Sage encyclopedia of qualitative research methods*. London/New Delhi/Thousand Oaks, CA: Sage Publications, 848–53

Williams R (2014) Facebook's 71 gender options come to UK users. *The Telegraph*, 27 June. www.telegraph.co.uk/technology/facebook/10930654/Facebooks-71-gender-options-come-to-UK-users.html

Wilson M (2002) 'I am the prince of pain, for I am a princess in the brain': liminal transgender identities, narratives and the elimination of ambiguities. *Sexualities* 5: 425–48

Women and Equalities Committee (2015) Transgender equality meeting, 8 September. http://parliamentlive.tv/event/index/7a72e9e0-ccee-4c46-9c5c-683d9a32fba7?

Wylie K, Barrett J, Besser M, et al. (2014) Good practice guidelines for the assessment and treatment of adults with gender dysphoria. *Sexual and Relationship Therapy* 29: 154–214

Wynn N (2018) Incels | ContraPoints. [Video] 17 August. www.youtube.com/watch?v=fD2briZ6fB0

Yeadon-Lee T (2016) What's the story? Exploring online narratives of non-binary gender identities. *The International Journal of Interdisciplinary Social and Community Studies* 11: 19–34

Ziegler K (2018) The peculiarity of black trans male privilege. In: Kimmel MS and Ferber AL (eds) *Privilege: A reader* (4th edn). London: Routledge

Zinn MB (1979) Field research in minority communities: ethical, methodological and political observations by an insider. *Social problems* 27: 209–19

Index

n = note